# Good Fats, Bad Fats

## Rosemary Stanton

ALLEN & UNWIN

*For all those who think fat is a foe.*

First published in 1997 by
Allen & Unwin
9 Atchison Street
St Leonards NSW 2065
Australia
Phone:  (61 2) 9901 4088
Fax:      (61 2) 9906 2218
E-mail:  frontdesk@allen-unwin.com.au
URL:     http://www.allen-unwin.com.au

National Library of Australia
Cataloguing-in-Publication entry:

Stanton, Rosemary.
  Good fats, bad fats.

  ISBN 1 86448 318 0.

  1. Fat. 2. Low-fat diet. I. Title.

613.284

Set in 10/11.5pt Palatino by DOCUPRO, Sydney
Printed and bound in Australia by Australian Print Group,
Maryborough, Victoria

10 9 8 7 6 5 4 3 2

# Contents

# Introduction

For some people, the word 'fat' conjures up images of rolls of flesh. Others think of fat in terms of greasy foods, deep-fryers or sausages. It would be good if we had separate words for different kinds of fat but we use the term for fats in food as well as for the fats that pad the body. They are intimately related because eating too many fatty foods leads to an increase in body fat. However, just as we all need some body fat, so we all need some food fats.

In Western countries, most people consume vast quantities of fatty foods. As a result, in countries such as Australia, half the men, about one-third of the women and approximately a quarter of the children have excessive deposits of body fat. Some overweight people accept that they have too much body fat, although others—especially some men—deny it. Many young women recoil from fat as if it were poison. Some suffer from total fat phobia, hating every hint of softness on their bodies and shunning fats in food as much as possible.

Others try to avoid food fats because they fear cancer, heart disease, stroke or diabetes. An excess of any kind of fat can lead to excess weight but the kind of fat is relevant for every other undesirable possibility linked with fat. Not all fats are equal. Yet few people distinguish between different types of fat.

Of those who continue to consume vast quantities of the stuff, some don't worry about fats at all. Others eat fats unwittingly because they have little idea which foods contain fat and how much fat some foods contain. The food industry makes this easy. In countries such as Australia, there is no legal requirement for food labels to state the fat level of the contents. Some companies do not even know how much fat their products contain, or are unwilling to publicise such information. Others confuse the issue with red herrings, such as the words 'no cholesterol', on the label. The food may have no cholesterol—a point of minor importance—but may still be stuffed with fat.

Many modern foods have more fat than their old-fashioned counterparts. Even a simple hamburger is deceiving. The kind of hamburgers once available, which often seemed quite greasy, averaged about 18 grams of fat. A modern burger, which does not seem to ooze much fat, has at least one and a half times as much fat, sometimes even more.

Large quantities of fats are also hidden in

unexpected places. For example, who would guess that a 70 gram croissant would have as much fat as nineteen slices of bread, that some cracker biscuits have twice the percentage of fat as lamingtons, or that crisps labelled 'light' would have more fat than their traditional counterparts.

The food industry has given us an enormous range of foods that are high in fat, and most of this fat is a type which nutritionists regard as undesirable. Even foods such as poly or mono-unsaturated margarine, which sound as though they have 'good' fats, also contain a lot of saturated or 'bad' fats. The food industry is now trying to make amends—or perhaps just greater profit—by producing an ever-expanding range of foods with reduced fat levels. These are among the fastest-growing lines. Many have less fat than the parent foods which spawned them, but they may still contain high levels. There is also a rapidly swelling range of fake fats. Some are already being used; others are still on the drawing board. Huge energy resources are being poured into producing fake food ingredients that will supply no energy. In a world where millions of people are starving, it seems almost obscene for wealthy nations to use energy resources and technology in this way. Their overfed populations can then stuff themselves with even more food, while others continue to starve for lack of food. To add insult to injury, when fake fats are excreted, many are not easily broken down and therefore add to pollution.

Discussing the issue of fats in food is not simple. Not all fats are equal and not all fats are undesirable. Some are essential. There are also serious doubts about the healthiness of some of the fake fats. We need to sort out the facts and understand which fats are beneficial, which are undesirable, how much of each type is safe and how we can achieve a balance between what our tastebuds want and our bodies need.

We also need to understand where different fats are found and which foods contribute the best balance of fats. By understanding the different types of fat—saturated, poly and mono-unsaturated, trans fatty acids, cholesterol, omega 3s and omega 6s—we may be able to choose fats wisely and dispel the idea that all fats are bad. Perhaps more important, our tastebuds may benefit from greater knowledge of the importance of quality and freshness in the fats we eat.

# CHAPTER 1

# The role of fat

## GENERAL VIEWS ABOUT FAT IN THE BODY

Until this century, most people thought body fat was good because it represented survival. They also thought highly of foods that contained fat, realising that those who could afford to eat more of these foods had higher stores of body fat, which was then available to supply energy for the body. In times when foods were scarce, or during illness, a store of fat could mean the difference between survival and death.

The idea that fat is good persists in many areas of the world, especially where an ample food supply is not always assured. In these parts, people still encourage young children to eat more, believing that a plump child is a sign of health and good parenting. In some societies, men consider that higher levels of body fat—or better still, a plump wife—demonstrate their wealth and worth as providers.

Some men in developed countries also believe that the sheer physical space a large, overweight body occupies is an imposing display of power. By contrast, many women feel so insecure about their role that they want to be as thin as possible. In extreme cases, these women develop eating disorders which are partly related to their intense fear of being fat.

In most parts of the world, however, there is a widespread belief that well-rounded women are more attractive, possibly because they are generally more fertile and fertility is still prized. The fecundity of well-rounded breasts and hips, and ample thighs, is a major reason why many great painters of the past have preferred to portray plumper women. Renoir, Reubens or Australia's Norman Lindsay would probably have pitied the supermodels of the 1990s for their lankiness and lack of flesh.

Up to a point, fatter women *are* more fertile, although this does not hold for the very obese who often suffer from infertility. Most women who are naturally lean are not infertile but many of those who reduce their normal body size to become as thin as current fashion demands will stop producing the female hormone oestrogen. This is nature's way of preventing pregnancy in a body that does not have enough fat stores to support a healthy pregnancy and period of lactation.

Endocrinologists tell us that girls begin to menstruate when their body fat reaches a level great enough to stimulate an increase in oestrogen production. As evidence for this, most plump girls menstruate early, whereas girls who are thinner may not begin menstruation until they are older. Those who are very thin may not menstruate at all.

Others believe menstruation begins when a girl's weight reaches a certain percentage of its genetically destined level, but this theory also depends partly on levels of body fat. All agree that linear growth slows once menstruation begins, when fat deposits develop on breasts, hips and thighs and the girl matures into womanhood. In a society obsessed with thinness and in which models are praised for their pre-pubescent low levels of body fat, some girls with normal fat deposits see themselves as having unsightly, abnormal fat bulges. Many think there is something wrong with their bodies and develop a dissatisfaction that can dominate their lives, leading to poor eating habits and low self-esteem. Most reject dietary fat when it comes from sources such as meat and dairy products, although they may continue to nibble on much fattier foods such as chips and chocolate.

The definition of anorexia nervosa includes the cessation of menstrual periods. Even when the psychological problems that are part of anorexia nervosa have improved, a girl is considered out of danger only when her body fat and oestrogen levels are high enough for her menstrual periods to return. From a physiological viewpoint, women need obvious deposits of body fat.

The structural components of the human body include bone, muscle and fat. Fat makes up about 15 per cent of the body weight of a normally sized man, and about 27 per cent of the weight of a normal woman. These are typical levels and some people are naturally leaner, while others may have higher levels of body fat.

The fat is present as essential fats in bone marrow and in organs such as the heart, spleen, kidneys, lungs, pancreas, brain and kidneys. The body's nervous system is also rich in essential fats. Women have about four times as much essential body fat as men because of their fat deposits on breasts, hips and thighs. These are considered as essential for women because of their role in fertility.

Both men and women also have extra deposits of storage fat in adipose tissue. Some of this is important to protect organs such as the kidneys, and to provide some degree of cushioning over the body. Most is stored beneath the skin as subcutaneous fat. About 12 per cent of men's body weight and 15 per cent of women's weight is storage fat. This fat also acts as insulation against the cold and those with less of it often feel the cold more intensely, although other factors, such as metabolic rate, are also important to protect the body against cold weather.

We need to stop thinking of all body fat as undesirable. Some is essential. Body fat is only a problem when levels are excessive and the fat is distributed as visceral fat around the abdomen. This occurs in men of all ages and post-menopausal women when they eat more than their body is burning for activity. Body fat is essential for normal bone density, especially in women. The risks associated with too little body fat and the problems of an excess of abdominal fat, and the food fats that contribute to it, are discussed in more detail in chapter 4.

## FAT IN FOOD—HISTORICAL PERSPECTIVE

From an historical perspective, problems due to excess body fat are recent but parallel the increase in foods rich in fat and the decrease in the amount of physical activity. If we go back to earlier times, or to the few remaining areas where people still live in more original conditions, it is easy to see why foods that contain fat are highly prized. They are rare. Wild animals have little body fat and virtually the only rich sources of fat are some animal organs such as the liver or brain, as well as the eggs of birds or turtles, nuts, seeds, and some grubs such as the witchetty grubs and

Bogong moths loved by the Aborigines. Animal flesh, most fish and other foods from the sea or rivers, native grasses, roots, tubers and wild fruits and vegetables have little fat. The mutton bird of the southern parts of Australia, or whales, seals and other creatures in polar regions are exceptions, but their fat is an interesting kind which is rich in omega 3 fatty acids.

In primitive societies, fat in large quantities is hard to find. For this reason, when an animal was killed, the brain and liver were so highly regarded that they were reserved for the most important members of the tribe. Such foods caused no problems because the total diet was so low in fat. The relatively high fat content of some fish, reptiles, moths and grubs did not contribute much total fat overall, because such foods were not eaten excessively, except in the Arctic circle where the diet was high in fat.

Essential fatty acids are found in the fats of nuts, seeds, eggs, and in most river, lake and saltwater foods. Grasses, wild vegetables and the lean flesh of animals, birds and reptiles also boost the intake of essential fatty acids, even though these foods contain only relatively small quantities of fat. Foods such as chocolate, crisps, chips and fried foods, on the other hand, have a lot of fat but little or no essential fatty acids.

In general, before animals were domesticated and packaged processed foods were readily available, only about 10 per cent of the day's energy came from fat. In most affluent countries, fat intake is now about four times this level, supplying about 40 per cent of energy. Average total energy intake in affluent countries has not increased to any extent, but its composition has changed dramatically from being high in carbohydrate to being high in fat.

Many populations, such as Australian Aborigines who have had few sources of fat in their diet, enjoy the flavour of foods that are rich in fat, especially fatty meats that may be rejected by other members of the population as being too fatty. When such foods were rare, they caused no problems. Unfortunately, very fatty meats are the cheapest types available, and many displaced people on low incomes, such as Aborigines, may consume enough of these meats for them to be a health hazard, contributing to high levels of diabetes and coronary heart disease.

Only the Inuit people (Eskimos), who once consumed large quantities of fatty cold-water fish, whales and seals, have a natural food supply that is rich in fat. Living in extremely cold conditions, this dietary fat was essential to increase body fat levels to provide insulation against the harsh weather conditions. The fats from these cold-water sea creatures are also rich in particular types of omega 3 polyunsaturated fatty acids, which may protect against heart disease and some cancers.

In stark contrast to the food supply available throughout millions of years of history over most parts of the earth, the modern Western food supply is saturated with vast quantities of fat. In the 1990s, separated fats, shortenings and margarines are the major sources of dietary fat. Most of these fats are added to foods such as fast foods and takeaways, crisps, chips, confectionery, biscuits, pastries, cakes and fried foods before we buy them. Meat is the next major source of fat, followed by dairy products. Contrary to popular belief, eggs do not contribute much fat, providing less than 2 per cent of the fat in the Australian diet.

In parts of Asia and the Middle East, fat consumption is also increasing rapidly, in line with affluence. Health authorities preach the virtues of eating more peasant-style food, with less fat, but in every society, as people become more affluent, they discard their healthy low-fat food habits for processed convenience foods. For example, in Japan, fat intake has accelerated over the last 20 years, rising from 10 per cent of energy to 25 per cent. Over the same period, subcutaneous body fat has more than doubled. Singaporeans show similar trends, and 25 per cent of the population now have excessively high levels of body fat, where once it was rare to find anyone in this category. Even in countries such as the United States, Europe or Australia, where there is a lot of adverse publicity about dietary fat and a plethora of fat-reduced foods, the fat intake continues to increase.

The increasing consumption of fatty fast foods and prepared takeaway foods, which now account for one third of the food dollar in Australia (even more in the United States), has been the major factor in the increasing fat consumption. Including fat-reduced dairy products and other low-fat products cannot make up for this massive influx of fat from fast foods.

The amount and sources of fat are not always apparent from surveys where individuals fill out questionnaires about how often they eat particular foods. Under such conditions, people tell you what they think you want to hear, not what they actually do. This distortion has increased over recent years when fat has had a bad press. Few people confess to a nutritionist how often they consume high-fat foods, so reports that people are eating less fat now than they were ten years ago reflect an increasing awareness of what one *should* eat, rather than the truth.

Women are still responsible for most food decisions, from shopping to cooking to cleaning up afterwards. Most women also have many other responsibilities in caring for home, children and aged relatives, and the majority work outside the home. Advertisers realise how processed and ready-prepared foods appeal to women. Their advertising reflects their desire to reduce the guilt that many women feel about using such products. There is not too much mystery, therefore, as to why people throughout the developed world have embraced processed and prepared foods. Many women know that fast foods are not as nutritious as good home cooking, so they do not accurately report how often they eat them. Sales figures, however, clearly indicate that consumption of fast foods, and consequently overall fat intake, is increasing.

Most people eat fast foods because they are cheap, convenient and save busy people the trouble of having to think about what to eat. They are also advertised heavily, and premises are clean and located to make visits easy and pleasant for children.

Few people eat these foods for the taste experience. Instead, most people's favourite food memories go back to their mother's home cooking, usually associated with good quality fresh ingredients mixed with a long session in the kitchen and a lot of love.

Old-style, home-cooked foods, however, were not fat free. Fat carries and develops flavour and all good cooks are aware of this. Frying is especially good at causing chemical changes which add to flavour. For example, you cannot get as much flavour by steaming an onion as you can when the onion is fried. But at least, when people cooked their foods from scratch, they were aware of the quantity of fat they included.

Few people are aware of the high fat content of foods someone else has prepared. The fact that processed and fast foods are high in fat is not a reason for purchase but an unfortunate coincidence. The misfortune relates to the type of fat such foods contain.

## FAT REQUIREMENTS

Fats from foods are essential to the body. They make up part of the structure of the membranes around all body cells and are important components of nerve and brain cells. Cholesterol, a type of waxy fat, is a precursor of sex and adrenal hormones, and is also needed to make bile acids used for the digestion of fats. Some fatty acids, known as essential fatty acids or EFAs, influence the body's production of prostaglandins, which have many hormone-like actions throughout body tissues. As well, fats provide an excellent source of kilojoules of energy.

Some fat from food is also converted into body fat. It cushions organs, gives padding to bones and joints and has the pleasing aesthetic purpose of giving a softer, more curved appearance. A small amount of body fat is also useful as a source of stored energy which can be used if food is unavailable, or during unexpected illness. Any kind of dietary fat can serve these purposes of increasing body fat, as all fats provide plenty of kilojoules of energy. The composition of cell membranes and body fat, however, can be influenced by the types of fats consumed. For example, eating a lot of saturated fat gives harder cell membranes and more solid body fat than occurs when the dietary fat is more unsaturated (see chapter 2).

With the best knowledge available at present, we assume that every gram of fat contributes 37 kilojoules, a level more than twice that for carbohydrates (which supply 16 kilojoules per gram) or protein (with 17 kilojoules per gram). Each gram of pure alcohol contributes 29 kilojoules.

Fats are made up of fatty acids and some researchers think that each gram of certain saturated fatty acids may contribute even more than 37 kilojoules. At this stage, however, 37 kilojoules is the accepted figure for all fats. As described in chapter 2, some fatty acids should have a greater role in the daily diet than others, but all fats are high in kilojoules. This is one reason why a diet high in fat easily leads to excess body weight.

A baby's first food is breast milk. It is a relatively high-fat food, supplying more than half its kilojoules of energy from fat. Most infants triple their birth weight in the first 12 to 15 months of life, and such a rapid growth rate needs the concentrated source of kilojoules that fat can provide.

Once growth stops, and certainly by the time we reach adulthood, we need much less dietary fat. The exact percentage of our energy that should come from fat is not certain. Before animals were domesticated to provide milk and meat, and long before processed foods dominated the diet, most human populations got about 10 per cent of their energy from fat. That may well be an ideal level.

In Western countries, most health authorities recommend cutting the fat content of the diet from its current level of about 40 per cent of energy to 30 per cent. No study has ever shown this figure to be optimal; it is set as a goal because it is considered to be potentially achievable within the food environment of developed countries.

We can make out a good case, however, that there is no *single* desirable level of dietary fat. The longest life expectancy occurred in Greece up to the 1960s. The Greek diet up to that time had at least 45 per cent of its kilojoules from fat. By contrast, the longest-living people in the 1990s are the Japanese and their diet has approximately 25 per cent of energy from fat, although most of the old people who are contributing to the statistics for long life expectancy would have had even lower levels of fat (approximately 15 per cent of energy) for most of their lives. It is also worth noting that the Greeks lived longer up to the 1960s than the Japanese do now. Since the Greeks reduced their total fat intake and substituted more saturated fats and processed foods for their previously olive oil-dominated diet, their incidence of coronary heart disease has increased and their length of life has decreased.

There seems to be much better evidence that it is not the *quantity* of fat that is important, but the *quality*. We also need to consider other protective factors from foods which may be making the major contribution to low death rates from both heart disease and cancers.

The Greek diet was rich in monounsaturated fat, mainly from olive oil and nuts. Both these foods are also rich in a wide variety of antioxidants which prevent the harmful effects produced when fats oxidise (see chapter 2 for more details). Fruits, vegetables, legumes, red wine and tea are also excellent sources of protective substances. Except for red wine, the Japanese diet and most other healthy diets contain plenty of these protective plant-based foods.

By contrast, the modern Western diet is rich in saturated fats, which we know can lead to fatty deposits in the arteries. Over the past few years, the content of polyunsaturated fats has also risen. These fats are essential in small quantities, but can oxidise readily in the arteries (and in the frying pan), causing damage. A very high level of polyunsaturates can also reduce levels of the 'good' cholesterol in blood, although this effect does not occur with a more moderate intake.

The idea that all body fat and fats in food are inherently bad is wrong. Body fat is not all bad and its relationship with healthiness follows a J-shape: those who are too thin or too fat are at greater risk of health problems. Among children, there is also plenty of evidence that fats from foods containing other nutrients necessary for growing children should not be shunned. For example, a low-fat diet in childhood is accompanied by low levels of pre-formed vitamin A. A lack of dietary fat also reduces the absorption of beta carotene, which the body can convert into vitamin A in older children and adults. This is a major reason why young children should be given regular milk rather than skim milk, which lacks both vitamin A and fat. Skim milk is fine for older children and adults who do not rely on milk as a major source of nutrients.

Elderly people may also need more dietary fat. Wasting is a problem of the very old, and a good source of kilojoules, such as fat, may help prevent it. It may therefore be inappropriate to tell the whole community to eat less fat when at both extremes of age the kilojoules fat supplies play a vital role. At these times, nutrient requirements may also be very high. It makes sense, therefore, for the very young and the very old to consume foods that supply fats along with other nutrients. This rules out promoting fatty chips, crisps, pastries, many fast foods and deep-fried products, pastries, biscuits and cakes as good foods for children or the elderly. High-fat but nutritious foods such as avocado, nuts or nut butters, seeds, fatty fish, eggs, good quality meats, milk, cheese and yoghurt would be more suitable.

The content of essential fatty acids in any fat is always important. The visible fat on meat and the fats used in most processed foods are low in essential fatty acids, whereas other foods that don't appear fatty at all, such as vegetables, may be important sources of essential fats.

Essential fatty acids contribute to the structure of the walls around every cell in the body, and are especially important to cells within the brain and nervous system. The term 'essential fatty acids' is used for those that cannot be made in the body and must be supplied from food.

One essential fatty acid is called linoleic acid and it belongs in the class of omega 6 fats (explained in chapter 2). There are also omega 3 fatty acids that are essential, but here we may have a choice. Alpha linolenic acid (often called ALA) is generally considered essential. It is found in some seeds especially linseeds, nuts, soy beans and vegetables and is converted in the body to eicosapentaenoic acid (EPA) and docosahexaenoic acid (DHA). These two fatty acids are found in freshwater and saltwater fish, and in mutton birds. These foods are therefore excellent substitutes for ALA. Breast milk is particularly rich in DHA which goes to the retina of the eye and the brain. Studies show that babies who are breastfed have sharper vision for the first eight or nine months of life, compared with those given formula milks.

## THE FUNCTIONS OF FAT IN FOOD

Fatty acids and other forms of fat are essential in the human body. Fatty acids, phospholipids and cholesterol form part of the structure of the membrane around every cell in the body. Phospholipids are also involved in blood clotting and cholesterol is needed for making bile for digestion and for the absorption of fats. Cholesterol is also needed to make some hormones, including sex hormones.

Fat is also needed to form body fat which cushions organs such as the kidneys, protects joints and serves as an important energy store. In moderate quantities, fat also adds pleasing curves to the human body. The functions of body fat are described further in chapter 4.

We can summarise the functions of fat in food as follows:

- To provide kilojoules, especially important for babies, the elderly and in any diseases where wasting may occur.
- To supply essential fatty acids which are used in cell membranes, in nerve, brain and skin cells and also in the retina of the eye, and for making prostaglandins (hormone-like substances that are involved in controlling inflammation, blood pressure and other body reactions).
- To make hormones (a specific function of cholesterol).
- To help the absorption of beta carotene (one type of carotenoid) which the body converts to vitamin A.
- To help the absorption of other carotenoids which are valuable in preventing many cancers.
- Fats delay the emptying of the stomach, giving a feeling of fullness after eating. While this can be an undesirable feature of an exceptionally fatty meal, it helps regulate the release of food from the stomach into the small intestine over several hours after a meal, preventing rapid return of hunger.
- To make body fat, needed for cushioning and insulation.

Fats may also accompany other important nutrients and protective factors in foods—for example, in nuts, avocado, seeds, soy beans, olive oil, fatty fish and yoghurt. Avoiding these foods because of their fat content could therefore have adverse effects.

Fats in foods also carry flavour. This is vitally important as flavoursome foods are more likely to be consumed. If you try to cook without any fat, few people will enjoy the food for long. For example, you cannot get the same flavour from a steamed or boiled onion as you do when you fry the onion in some oil. Nor will low-fat ice-cream have as much creamy taste as regular or premium ice-cream or low-fat cheese seriously rival full-fat cheese.

The fact that fats bring out and carry flavour does not mean you need to eat vast quantities of fat to have good-tasting foods. For example, the onion fried in two teaspoons of oil will have just as much flavour as one cooked in two tablespoons of oil.

# CHAPTER 2
# Types of fat

Some of the information in this chapter is included for those seeking more detailed information about fats and their role in food. If some paragraphs seem too complicated, please skip to the following one.

## THE STRUCTURE OF FATS

Fats in foods are more properly called 'lipids' and consist of a mixture of different substances including triglycerides (also called triacylglycerols), phospholipids, sterols such as cholesterol, waxes, lipoproteins (combinations of fat and protein) and other related compounds. To discuss fats more fully, we need to describe some aspects of their chemistry.

Triglycerides are the most common fats and make up more than 95 per cent of body fat. They consist of a basic framework of a backbone molecule of glycerol, which is chemically an alcohol comprising three carbon atoms combined with three hydroxyl (OH) groups to which are attached three fatty acids. Glycerol comprises about 10 per cent of the weight of this framework. Without any fatty acids attached, glycerol itself is sometimes used in icing and confectionery to stop sugar molecules crystallising. It is also used in lipstick. Various di- and mono-glycerides are used in place of fats in fat-reduced products, as discussed in chapter 5.

Fatty acids consist of a chain of carbon atoms, with three hydrogen atoms attached to the carbon atom at one end (known as the methyl end), and an oxygen atom and a hydroxyl group (OH) attached to the last carbon at the other end (known as the hydroxyl or carboxylic acid end). There can be as many as 35 carbon atoms in the chain, although the most common fatty acids have between 4 and 22 carbon atoms.

The three fatty acids in a triglyceride attach at the hydroxyl (or acidic) end of their molecules, losing their hydroxyl group in the process. They can be arranged in different ways on the glycerol backbone of the molecule and may rearrange themselves during processing. For example, fatty acids present in an oil may change position if the oil is processed into mayonnaise or margarine. The arrangement of the fatty acids influences physical characteristics such as the melting point of the processed product.

Most triglycerides have a saturated fatty acid at position 1 on the glycerol molecule and an unsaturated fatty acid at position 2. The third position varies. Triglycerides that contain at least two saturated fatty acids are usually solid at room temperature whereas those with two unsaturated fatty acids are oils at room temperature.

Some medical researchers have also found that changes in the arrangement of the fatty acids may alter the way the fat is used in the body. If future research confirms that this is important, such factors may be taken into account when giving advice about whether to eat processed or unprocessed fats.

Cold-pressed oils, made by squashing the oil-rich fruit of olives, the seeds of grapes or sunflowers, or legumes such as peanuts or soy beans, probably retain their original and most desirable arrangement of fatty acids, along with their rich supply of different anti-oxidants. Oils that are extracted with a chemical solvent and processed into spreads, shortenings or frying fats may become rearranged and thereby lose some of their original anti-oxidants. At present, the way fats are produced is often ignored because no one is certain how important it is. Some argue that once fats are consumed, the first stage in digestion is to split the fatty acids away from the glycerol part of the molecule, making their original arrangement less important.

Oils extracted using a chemical solvent usually have an anti-oxidant added to stop them going rancid. The *quantity* of anti-oxidant in cold-pressed or solvent-extracted oils is similar but the cold-pressed products may have many anti-oxidants, rather than a single variety of added anti-oxidant. Again, no one can say for certain whether this matters but many researchers believe the real value of olive oil lies with its diversity of anti-oxidants as much as with the type of fatty acids it contains.

When fatty acids join onto a triglyceride, losing their acidic ends, they are referred to as 'fats'. This term includes products that are solid or liquid, although those that are liquid at room temperature are conventionally called oils. When nutritionists refer to the fat content of the diet, however, they include all types of fats and oils.

## SATURATION

Fatty acids vary in the type of chemical bonds between the carbon atoms in their chain. Usually each carbon atom uses two of its four bonds to hold onto the carbon atoms that lie either side of it in the carbon chain. The remaining two bonds each hold a hydrogen atom. When two adjacent carbon atoms each hold only one hydrogen atom, they can use their free 'hands' to double the bond between them, forming what is known as a *double bond*.

To simplify the task of classifying them, fatty acids are usually divided into classes of saturated, monounsaturated and polyunsaturated fats, according to the number and type of bonds the fatty acid contains. A saturated fatty acid has no double bonds in its chain, a monounsaturated fatty acid has only one double bond in its chain, while a polyunsaturated fatty acid has at least two. You may also hear these fatty acids referred to as saturates, mono-unsaturates and polyunsaturates.

## Saturated fats

A saturated fat has a straight carbon chain and no double bonds. This means that every carbon atom up to the last carbon atom in the chain has its bonds attached to a hydrogen atom. Because they have as many hydrogen atoms attached as possible, they are said to be 'saturated' (with hydrogen).

The saturated fatty acids are listed below, with the number of carbon atoms they contain and the way this is often abbreviated. For example, palmitic acid, one of the most common saturated fats, is written as C16:0, meaning that it has 16 carbon atoms in its chain and no double bonds. Stearic acid, another common saturated fatty acid, has 18 carbon atoms and is written as C18:0. Chocolate and red meats are major sources of palmitic and stearic acids.

Saturated fats are found in both animal and plant foods. Some people wrongly assume that they come only from animal sources. Vegetable foods such as coconut, palm oil, palm kernel oils and cocoa butter (used for making chocolate) are rich in saturated fats.

When vegetable fats and oils are processed into solid or spreadable fats for spreads or as shortenings for making pastries and cakes, some of those that were once largely unsaturated acquire extra hydrogen atoms to become saturated fats. This process is called hydrogenation. It increases the stability of the fat so that it does not go rancid so easily, but it also changes the nature of the fat to one that is much less desirable. When a food label lists 'hydrogenated vegetable oil' among the ingredients, the product will have a higher content of saturated fat than the original oil from which it was made. Many commercially fried foods claiming to have been cooked in vegetable oil have usually been cooked in a vegetable oil that was first hydrogenated into a saturated fat. Some of these fats are much higher in saturated fat than beef dripping or lard but consumers mistakenly believe they are better because the label describes them as 'vegetable'. There are also other fatty acids with odd numbers of carbon atoms but these occur less often in foods.

| Saturated fatty acids | No. of carbon atoms | Notation |
|---|---|---|
| Acetic acid | 2 | C2:0 |
| Propionic acid | 3 | C3:0 |
| Butyric acid | 4 | C4:0 |
| Caproic acid | 6 | C6:0 |
| Caprylic acid | 8 | C8:0 |

| Saturated fatty acids | No. of carbon atoms | Notation |
|---|---|---|
| Capric acid | 10 | C10:0 |
| Lauric acid | 12 | C12:0 |
| Myristic acid | 14 | C14:0 |
| Palmitic acid | 16 | C16:0 |
| Stearic acid | 18 | C18:0 |
| Arachnic acid | 20 | C20:0 |
| Behenic acid | 22 | C22:0 |
| Lignoceric acid | 24 | C24:0 |

Acetic acid is vinegar, not a product you would normally consider as 'fatty'. Acetic, propionic, butyric, caproic and caprylic acids are all soluble in water and none of them are 'fatty' in the usual sense of the word. In the technical language of chemists, however, they are fatty acids.

Acetic, propionic and butyric acids are usually found in the colon (bowel). They are made by bacteria that ferment dietary fibre, and butyric acid serves as a fuel for cells in the bowel. There is a growing body of evidence that butyric acid (also called butyrate) protects against bowel cancer.

Each of the fatty acids with up to eight carbon atoms in its chain is called a *short-chain* fatty acid, although some people consider that caprylic acid fits better as a medium-chain fatty acid. They are found only in small quantities in most foods.

Dairy products are the major source and butter has a high content of butyric acid, as its name suggests. Goat's milk has a high content of capric acid, with four to seven times as much of this fatty acid as human milk and about three times the level found in cow's milk.

Capric, lauric and (depending on your classification) caprylic acid are called *medium-chain* fatty acids and are found in a range of foods. Lauric acid is the major fatty acid in coconut. Some people also include myristic acid as a medium-chain fatty acid; others class it as long-chain.

Oils containing medium-chain triglycerides (MCT) are made from coconut oil and consist mainly of caprylic and capric saturated fatty acids. They are broken down by the body more easily than other triglycerides are, and once they are absorbed, the hepatic-portal vein blood carries them straight to the liver, where they can provide a quick source of energy, if needed. Until recently, most researchers assumed that medium-chain triglycerides had little effect on blood cholesterol, but recent studies show this is wrong.

Some sports people mistakenly assume that MCTs have advantages over other fats in providing a ready source of energy to enhance performance. There is no evidence to support this and nothing to justify the high prices sometimes charged for these fats. One study showed that

MCT oils can easily end up as abdominal fat. Most sports people need more carbohydrate to supply energy, not fat.

All the fatty acids with more than 14 carbon atoms are called *long-chain* fatty acids and they are the predominant type of saturated fat in most foods. High sources include almost all fast foods and takeaway items; most commercial fried foods; red meats; chicken; dairy products such as butter, cream, cheese, yoghurt, regular milk and margarine; processed foods such as pastries, cakes, biscuits (sweet and savoury); and chocolate. Myristic is coconut's second most common fatty acid and is also present in fairly high quantity in dairy products and in goat's milk.

Saturated fatty acids contribute energy and are important for growth in young animals and human babies. Too many saturated fats are undesirable, however, as they lead to an increase in blood cholesterol and blood clotting and are strongly correlated with coronary heart disease and adult-onset diabetes.

## Monounsaturated fats

The term 'unsaturated' fats includes monounsaturated and polyunsaturated fats. Monounsaturated fatty acids (sometimes referred to as MUFA) have two hydrogen atoms missing from a point in their carbon chain. The two carbon atoms then form what is called a 'double bond'. The position from the methyl end of the fatty acid is written as n–7 or n–9, which indicates that the double bond occurs on the seventh or ninth carbon (that is, between the seventh and eighth, or ninth and tenth carbon atoms respectively).

The most common monounsaturated fatty acid is oleic acid, and its major sources are olive, canola, peanut and macadamia oils, most nuts (except walnuts and pecans), avocado, fish, chicken and wild meats such as venison and kangaroo. Oleic acid is also the most widespread of all fatty acids, and is the most dominant type in all kinds of meat, eggs, dairy products, lard, dripping and all margarines, except those labelled 'polyunsaturated'.

| Monounsaturated fatty acids | No. of carbon atoms | | Notation |
|---|---|---|---|
| Palmitoleic acid | 16 | | C16:1 n–7 |
| Oleic acid | 18 | (cis) | C18:1 n–9 |
| Elaidic acid | 18 | (trans) | C18:1 n–9 |
| Eicosenoic | 20 | | C20:1 |
| Erucic acid | 22 | | C22:1 n–9 |
| Cetoleic acid | 22 | | C22:1 n–11 |

Erucic acid comes from rapeseeds, a vegetable crop that grows easily and crops heavily. Unfortunately, erucic acid enters the cells, including those in the heart muscle, and accumulates there due to its very slow rate of oxidation. This is so undesirable that no oil sold in Europe or the UK may contain more than 5 per cent erucic acid. Plant geneticists have developed a rapeseed with only 2 per cent erucic acid which is now sold as canola oil. Its fatty acid pattern has mainly oleic acid but also some alpha-linolenic acid. Theoretically, it looks even better than olive oil, although it does not have the history of use, the flavour or variety of anti-oxidants found in olive oil.

Monounsaturated fatty acids are generally considered the 'good guys' because they do not increase blood cholesterol levels. The exception is elaidic acid, a fatty acid formed when polyunsaturated fats are processed to make spreads. Elaidic acid is called a trans fatty acid because of the way its molecule lies. It does not occur in nature.

## Polyunsaturated fats

Polyunsaturated fatty acids (sometimes called PUFA) have more than one double bond between carbon atoms in their chain. They fit into two major classes: omega 6, written as n–6; and omega 3, written as n–3. These terms refer to the position of the first double bond from the methyl end of the molecule. Thus an omega 6 fatty acid has its first double bond on the sixth carbon from the methyl end of the molecule, while omega 3s have the first double bond on the third carbon atom.

These basic fatty acids are converted in the body to hormone-like substances called prostaglandins, thromboxanes and prostacyclins. The omega 3 and 6 positions are important because the types of prostaglandins made from each have opposite, but potentially complementary, roles. Too much of one kind in relation to the quantity of the other can alter inflammatory reactions in the body's tissues and interfere with the stickiness of blood cells, changing how much or how little blood cells will form clots.

In the modern Western diet, the ratio of omega 6 to omega 3 fatty acids has become unbalanced, largely because of a greatly increased consumption of an omega 6 polyunsaturated fatty acid called linoleic acid. This fatty acid is essential in small quantities, which is how it would normally be consumed in a diet of natural wholefoods.

Omega 3 fatty acids have a more limited distribution in the food chain and the balance between the two types has suffered as a result. Vegetables, some seeds, canola and soy bean oils contain small quantities of an omega 3 fatty acid called alpha-linolenic acid, while fish and other seafoods and breast milk are excellent sources of very long-chain omega 3s.

Linoleic acid is the major polyunsaturated fatty acid in Western diets. Intake has risen steadily as polyunsaturated margarines and oils have become more popular. Major sources include margarines and vegetable oils such as corn, safflower, sunflower, soy bean, cottonseed, grapeseed and sesame. Walnuts, pecans and Brazil nuts have more polyunsaturated fat than other nuts, which are higher in monounsaturated fatty acids.

| Polyunsaturated fatty acids | No. of carbon atoms | Notation |
|---|---|---|
| Linoleic acid | 18 | C18:2 n–6 |
| Alpha-linolenic acid | 18 | C18:3 n–3 |
| Gamma-linolenic acid | 18 | C18:3 n–6 |
| Dihomo-gamma-linolenic acid | 20 | C20:3 n–6 |
| Eicosatrenoic acid | 20 | C20:3 n–9 |
| Stearidonic acid | 18 | C18:4 n–3 |
| Arachidonic acid | 20 | C20:4 n–6 |
| Eicosatetraenoic acid | 20 | C20:4 n–3 |
| Docosatetraenoic (or adrenic acid) | 22 | C22:4 n–6 |
| Eicosapentaenoic acid (EPA) | 20 | C20:5 n–3 |
| Docosapentaenoic acid | 22 | C22:5 n–6 |
| Docosapentaenoic acid | 22 | C22:5 n–3 |
| Docosahexaenoic acid (DHA) (or clupanodonic acid) | 22 | C22:6, n–3 |

## ESSENTIAL FATTY ACIDS (EFAs)

The body must have some essential long-chain fatty acids: arachidonic acid, an omega 6 fatty acid; and the omega 3 fatty acids, EPA (eicosapentaenoic acid) and DHA (docosahexaenoic acid).

These fatty acids are involved in growth, and are vital for making hormone-like substances called prostaglandins, which in turn are required for making prostacyclins and thromboxanes. These compounds make blood clot enough but not too much, and also influence inflammatory reactions in tissues, blood pressure, the reproductive cycle, pain sensations, uterine contractions during labour, and many other functions. DHA is also important in infancy (it is present in breast milk), as well as in the retina of the eye and in the brain. Infants who are breastfed have much sharper vision for the first few months of life than those who are given formula milks.

The essential omega 6 and omega 3 fatty acids must be in balance with each other. For example, too much of the omega 6s relative to omega 3s will make blood clot too readily whereas the opposite will allow excessive bleeding after a cut. This was first noticed in the Inuit people, who have a very high intake of omega 3 fatty acids from fish, seal flesh and whale blubber. They did not have clots forming in their arteries and blocking blood vessels but they bled for a long time after a cut.

Essential fatty acids have very long carbon chains and can be made in the body from the parent compounds—linoleic acid (LA) and alpha-linolenic acid (ALA). Enzymes gradually elongate the molecule, adding more carbon atoms. The sequence of fatty acids is shown below. For the most commonly discussed acids, the initials by which they are commonly known are written in brackets.

**Fatty acid pathways**

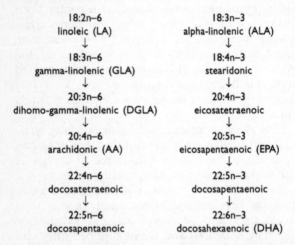

| | |
|---|---|
| 18:2n–6<br>linoleic (LA)<br>↓ | 18:3n–3<br>alpha-linolenic (ALA)<br>↓ |
| 18:3n–6<br>gamma-linolenic (GLA)<br>↓ | 18:4n–3<br>stearidonic<br>↓ |
| 20:3n–6<br>dihomo-gamma-linolenic (DGLA)<br>↓ | 20:4n–3<br>eicosatetraenoic<br>↓ |
| 20:4n–6<br>arachidonic (AA)<br>↓ | 20:5n–3<br>eicosapentaenoic (EPA)<br>↓ |
| 22:4n–6<br>docosatetraenoic<br>↓ | 22:5n–3<br>docosapentaenoic<br>↓ |
| 22:5n–6<br>docosapentaenoic | 22:6n–3<br>docosahexaenoic (DHA) |

Breast milk, the 'gold standard' food for humans, has about five times as many omega 6 fatty acids as omega 3s. A ratio of up to 6:1 is considered acceptable for adults. However, the modern Western diet that includes polyunsaturated oils and margarines, which are rich in linoleic acid, may have 14 to 40 times as much omega 6 as omega 3 fatty acids. Those who eat fish several times a week will have a more favourable ratio because fish and seafoods have ready-made long-chain essential omega 3 fatty acids.

For those who do not eat fish, and therefore rely on making the essential EPA and DHA from alpha-linolenic acid, an excess of linoleic acid is a problem. Alpha-linolenic acid is regarded as 'essential' because it can be used to make the longer-chain fats, but to do this it requires the same enzyme for the first stage of chain elongation as linoleic acid does. If linoleic acid is present in large quantities, it will preferentially 'use up' this enzyme, thus preventing alpha-linolenic acid being converted to the final essential fatty acids. Oils such as canola advertise their content of omega 3 fatty acid as a selling point. This is present as alpha-linolenic acid, however, and is useful only if the diet does not also contain a lot of polyunsaturated products.

The easiest solution to these problems is to use an omega 9 oil, such as olive, in preference to a polyunsaturated oil, and to eat plenty of vegetables as well as fish or other seafoods regularly. Olive oil does not enter the competition and so does not prevent the alpha-linolenic acid in vegetables being converted to the truly essential longer-chain fatty acids. The omega 6 fatty acids are present in much larger quantities and a deficiency is a problem only for those who try to avoid all fats.

## PROSTAGLANDINS AND EICOSANOIDS

Eicosanoids is a general term that embraces substances called prostaglandins, thromboxanes and leukotrienes which have hormone-like actions in the body. Since they control blood pressure, blood clotting, the reproductive cycle and inflammatory reactions, they are vital for health and are made from the fatty acids dihomo-gamma-linolenic acid (DGLA), arachidonic acid (AA) and eicosapentaenoic acid (EPA). These in turn are made from linoleic acid and alpha-linolenic acid, the two fatty acids called 'essential' fatty acids.

Arachidonic acid also occurs in turkey, meat and fish. DGLA can be made from evening primrose oil, blackcurrant or borage seed oils, and EPA can be obtained from fish or from stearidonic acid which is found in blackcurrant oil.

The thromboxanes and leukotrienes derived from the omega 3 and omega 6 fatty acids must be in balance or blood clotting and inflammatory reactions may be adversely affected. For arthritis, an inflammation of the joints, and also for people whose blood clots too readily, more of the omega 3 fatty acids and less of the omega 6s can help. In practice, this means eating more fish and vegetables, and less margarine and polyunsaturated vegetable oils.

## EVENING PRIMROSE OIL

This fatty acid is high in gamma-linolenic acid (GLA), an omega 6 fatty acid, and is often promoted as an essential supplement. It has some uses, especially for children who lack the enzyme delta-6-desaturase, which is needed to make GLA from linoleic acid. Such children may develop a particular type of eczema in early infancy. Until their bodies begin to produce adequate amounts of the enzyme, a regular supplement of evening primrose oil, with its high content of GLA, can help their eczema. Since only a few forms of eczema are related to GLA, only a few can be helped by supplements of evening primrose oil.

Many women also take evening primrose oil for menopausal or pre-menopausal problems although there is no proof that it has any greater effect than a placebo (dummy capsule).

It is hard to understand the rationale for prescribing evening primrose oil to a population that already has high levels of linoleic acid, which is converted to GLA, the major fat in evening primrose oil. The only rationale would be a lack of the delta-6-desaturase enzyme and there is no evidence of this. In fact, the type of prostaglandins that dominate blood clotting show that most people would be better off without so many omega 6 fatty acids. Borage and blackberry oils have even higher levels of GLA and are also promoted—at a high price.

Research into evening primrose oil and other oils rich in omega 6 fatty acids is continuing and they may turn out to have some unforeseen use. Some keen salespeople often try to sell evening primrose oil as a source of omega 3 fatty acids. You should question their knowledge of the subject of essential fatty acids.

## PHOSPHOLIPIDS

A glycerol molecule may also have two fatty acids attached (a diglyceride) plus a molecule of phosphoric acid attached to either inositol or a compound containing nitrogen, such as choline or serine. Inositol and choline are both members of the vitamin B complex but neither are regarded as vitamins or needed as supplements for humans as they can be made in the body. Serine is an amino acid that makes up part of proteins. Phospholipids are important in the structure of nerves and muscles.

Phospholipids are water soluble at one end and fat soluble at the other. This makes them excellent detergents. The best known is lecithin, commonly used as an emulsifier because it can link water and fat. Lecithin makes up about 30 per cent of an egg yolk and it is this property of egg yolk that can stop fat and water separating in products such as mayonnaise or Hollandaise sauce. Lecithin can also be extracted from soy beans and made into granules to sprinkle over breakfast cereals. As well, lecithin is widely used in processed foods to stop oily components separating out of foods such as sauces, dressings, mayonnaise, desserts and peanut butter. The human body makes its own lecithin to transport fats around the body, so that taking extra quantities, either as granules or in tablets, has no special benefit. Claims that taking lecithin will reduce cholesterol are unproven. It also has no effect in reducing body weight. Few people are likely to take enough of it to increase their weight, although it is a fat.

## CHOLESTEROL

This waxy fat belongs to a class of fats called sterols. In the body it forms an essential part of the structure of all cell membranes and is also used for making the bile acids necessary for the digestion and absorption of fats. It is also needed for making vitamin D and some hormones.

The body does not need a ready-made source of cholesterol as it can be made in the liver and in some body cells. When the diet is high in saturated fat, many people make more cholesterol than they need. In the body, cholesterol is carried through the blood attached to lipoproteins. If a high level of cholesterol is being carried on low-density lipoproteins (LDL), some cholesterol may be deposited in the walls of arteries, and if these deposits are in the coronary arteries and become oxidised, they break off in pieces known as foam cells. These can block the artery so that blood cannot get through, causing an infarction (heart attack).

Some anti-oxidants may prevent this oxidation reaction occurring. Products such as olive oil, which can have 30 to 40 different anti-oxidants, can help to prevent this reaction. Fruits, vegetables, nuts, red wine and tea are also excellent sources of protective anti-oxidants. The inclusion of olive oil and most of these foods in the diet may explain why people in Mediterranean countries have such low rates of coronary heart disease even though their average cholesterol levels are similar to those in populations in countries such as Australia and the United States.

Although about 80 per cent of the 100–150 grams of cholesterol in the body is made in the liver, some is also available, ready-made, from animal foods. A very high intake of these can increase blood cholesterol levels, but this usually occurs only when the diet is also high in saturated fat. People with high cholesterol levels are often told to avoid foods such as prawns or squid because they are high in cholesterol, but avoiding them is unnecessary because these foods have almost no saturated fat. In a few studies, volunteers have eaten large quantities of seafoods and found that there is no rise in their bad LDL cholesterol, although some have reported a favourable increase in good HDL cholesterol. From the serving sizes of prawns that most people could afford, it is fair to say they will have no effect on their blood cholesterol.

Egg yolks can raise cholesterol, but only if the diet is high in saturated fat. Eggs contribute about 1 per cent of the saturated fat in the Australian diet and can, for practical purposes, be ignored. If you ate daily helpings of fatty bacon and fried eggs served on buttered toast, your blood cholesterol levels would almost certainly increase because the ready-made cholesterol was being served with a hearty supply of saturated fat. Those whose blood cholesterol level is high should restrict saturated fats in the diet rather than foods containing cholesterol.

Many food labels proudly boast 'no cholesterol' claims. These are irrelevant and often misleading, especially when placed on foods that are high in saturated fat. In Australia, there are now guidelines for manufacturers recommending that 'no cholesterol' should appear only on foods that have less than 3 grams of fat per 100 grams.

Manufacturers who flout these guidelines are not currently penalised, however, and so there are many instances of confusion for consumers.

## The cholesterol content of foods

| Food | Cholesterol content (milligrams) |
| --- | --- |
| Egg, 1 | 210 |
| Ice-cream, 2 small scoops | 10 |
| Milk, 250 mL | 35 |
| Skim milk, 250 mL | 5 |
| Milk, mature breast, 250 mL | 40 |
| Colostrum, 100g | 30 |
| Butter, 1 tablespoon | 45 |
| Cheese, 30g slice | 30 |
| Cottage cheese, 50g | 5 |
| Yoghurt, 200g | 20 |
| Yoghurt, low-fat, 200g | 5 |
| Cream, 2 tablespoons | 40 |
| Cake, plain, average slice | 50 |
| Beef, cooked, lean & fat, 150g | 120 |
| Beef, cooked, lean only, 150g | 120 |
| Lamb, cooked, 150g | 165 |
| Pork, cooked, 150g | 165 |
| Chicken, cooked, 150g | 130 |
| Kidney, lamb, cooked, 100g | 610 |
| Kidney, ox, cooked, 100g | 690 |
| Liver, lamb, cooked, 100g | 400 |
| Liver, calf, cooked, 100g | 330 |
| Liver, chicken, cooked, 100g | 350 |
| Brains, cooked, 100g | 2600 |

| Food | Cholesterol content (milligrams) |
|---|---|
| Fish, grilled, 150g | 75 |
| Squid, cooked, 100g | 190 |
| Prawns, cooked, 100g flesh | 200 |
| Oysters, 12 | 60 |
| Mussels, 6 | 120 |

# THE DIGESTION OF FATS

A small amount of fat-splitting enzyme called lingual lipase is produced in the mouth. As fats are swallowed and pass to the stomach, this enzyme can begin splitting off one fatty acid from triglycerides. Virtually no other breakdown of fats occurs until fat reaches the small intestine where bile salts act as detergents and break the fats into small droplets. Enzymes (lipases) then split the fats into a mixture of free fatty acids, monoglycerides and diglycerides. Two of the fatty acids attached to the triglyceride are removed; the third, in position known as sn–2, remains attached to glycerol. Bile acids and phospholipids act as detergents and help the smaller particles of digested fats pass into the cells of the small intestine walls. The bile salts are left behind but almost all fat is absorbed.

Within the cells further splitting of fats occurs, then the fatty acids reform into new triglycerides. These are combined with proteins and incorporated into lipoproteins called chylomicrons which pass into the thoracic duct in the neck and thence into the bloodstream. Short-chain fatty acids and glycerol do not take this route but pass directly into the portal vein and go straight to the liver.

Chylomicrons are important to transport triglycerides, cholesterol and fat-soluble vitamins from the wall of the intestine to other parts of the body where they can be used or stored. The core of the chylomicron particle contains triglycerides and the surface carries phospholipids, cholesterol and compounds called apoproteins.

## THE TRANSPORT OF FATS IN THE BODY

Fats don't dissolve in water, so for transport in the blood they are combined with proteins. If they were not, they would float on top of the blood, as cream does in milk that has not been homogenised. In combination, proteins and fats are called lipoproteins and, in this form, fats can travel in blood. Depending on how closely the lipoproteins are packed together, they are called very low-density lipoproteins (VLDL), intermediate density (IDL), low-density (LDL) or high-density lipoproteins (HDL).

VLDLs consist of a little over 50 per cent triglycerides plus some phospholipids and cholesterol. They are formed in the liver, either from triglycerides made from sugars consumed in a meal or snack, or between meals from fats that have been mobilised from stored fat deposits in the body. VLDLs take triglycerides to the body's tissues, where they are used for energy or kept in storage. At this stage, the cholesterol component dominates the VLDL which increases in density to become an IDL which, in turn, loses some of its fats and becomes a low-density lipoprotein.

The major type of fat in LDL is cholesterol. Some of this is deposited in peripheral tissues and into arteries where it can build up into deposits called plaque.

HDL particles have about 45 per cent of their fat as phospholipids and can pick up cholesterol from the peripheral tissues, forming a compound called HDL3. This in turn picks up more cholesterol as well as some phospholipids and proteins from VLDL to form HDL2. Once HDL2 gets to the liver, it is broken down and the cholesterol is excreted or used for making bile and hormones.

LDL cholesterol in the blood is commonly called 'bad' cholesterol as it carries cholesterol to tissues such as the arteries. The level of LDL in the blood is strongly correlated with coronary heart disease. HDL cholesterol is known as 'good' cholesterol because it is a sign that cholesterol has been scavenged from the tissue and is being taken to the liver. A high level of HDL reduces the risk of coronary heart disease.

Another lipoprotein particle called Lp(a) increases the risk of cardiovascular disease. It is a genetic factor and high levels in the blood can double the risk of heart attack in men before age 55. Until recently, most people believed that Lp(a) could not be influenced by diet or other aspects of daily living, but it now appears that trans fatty acids in some margarines and processed fats can increase it. There is some evidence that red wine may decrease Lp(a).

## TRANS FATTY ACIDS

Some unsaturated fatty acids can have a kink at the site of the double bond in their carbon chain. Where a kink is present, the hydrogen atoms on adjacent carbon atoms may occur on the same or opposite side of the molecule. Those on the same side are said to be in a *cis* configuration; those with the hydrogen atoms opposite each other are called *trans* fats. The shape of a *cis* molecule allows it to double back on itself so that such fats can be more tightly packed into larger fats. In their natural state, both plant and animal foods have their unsaturated fatty acids in the *cis* form. The *trans* form develops mainly when fats are processed, although small amounts of some trans fatty acids are found in meat and dairy products.

The interest in trans fatty acids increased when medical researchers noted in several studies that one particular trans monounsaturated fatty acid with 18 carbon atoms, called *elaidic acid*, is nasty because it can reduce levels of 'good' cholesterol in the blood and raise levels of 'bad' cholesterol. It can also increase levels of a compound called lipoprotein(a) or Lp(a), which can then increase the risk of coronary heart disease.

Several studies reported a strong association between the level of trans fats ingested, mainly from margarine, and these risk factors for coronary heart disease. One major study of over 85,000 nurses in the United States found that those who had consumed plenty of foods high in elaidic acid (mainly margarine) had a 50 per cent greater risk of coronary heart disease than those who ate less margarine.

One major study did not support such findings. Researchers took samples of body fat from men who had already had a heart attack and also from control subjects. They collected samples from ten countries and analysed them to see if those who had suffered a heart attack had more trans fatty acids in their body fat than those who had remained healthy. They found no significant difference between the two groups, although this may have been due to their inability to distinguish between trans fatty acids that occur naturally and those produced by partial hydrogenation of oils. Levels of trans fats differed greatly between countries. The researchers did not rule out the possibility of a greater effect of trans fats on people in countries where the intake is high. Both groups from Spain had low levels of trans fats in their body fat, probably because their major dietary fat is olive oil, not margarine or processed fats. Spain has a very low level of coronary heart disease.

Medical research is difficult at the best of times, but research on dietary factors is especially so. One researcher has suggested that trans fatty acids may be harmful only when a person is consuming too many kilojoules. Enough studies have now suggested that they are undesirable and the food industry should exclude them from processed foods. They are not necessary and there are many better, though not necessarily cheaper, fats available.

Elaidic acid can form when polyunsaturated fatty acids from vegetable or fish oils are partly hydrogenated to form margarines and shortenings for processed and fast foods. The naturally occurring trans fatty acids in meat and dairy products do not have the same effect and so are not of concern. (These foods have a high content of saturated fatty acids which can cause other problems.)

In Australia, fish oils are not used in processed foods, but in the United Kingdom, Norway, the Netherlands and some other parts of Europe they are deodorised and processed into a shortening for pastries, pies, biscuits, hamburger rolls and other processed foods. The content of elaidic acid in these hydrogenated fats is high but they are used because they are cheap and the processed fats have a longer shelf life than natural fats do. Many nutritionists now consider them undesirable.

In areas of India and Pakistan, a partly hydrogenated vegetable oil called vanaspathi is used. It contains very high levels of elaidic acid, the trans fat. The *British Medical Journal* recently reported that areas where this type of fat is consumed have a high level of coronary heart disease.

Margarines can be produced with minimal quantities of elaidic acid but manufacturers are caught in a cleft stick. They can either make products containing elaidic acid, the undesirable trans fatty acid, or they can avoid it by increasing the level of saturated fatty acids—another undesirable feature.

Some margarine manufacturers have taken heed of the potentially adverse effects of this trans fat and are making their products with minimal quantities. Others believe the hazards have been overstated and so continue to sell polyunsaturated or monounsaturated margarines containing up to 15 per cent of elaidic acid. Unfortunately, countries such as Australia do not require food manufacturers to list the content of trans fatty acid, although organisations such as the National Heart Foundation have recommended it.

The problem for the margarine manufacturers is how to rank fatty acids according to which are the most undesirable. The problem for the consumer lies in knowing which is the best of a bad lot. The best solution may be to skip yellow fats as much as possible.

Of even greater concern is the trend towards using hardened canola and cottonseed oils in processed foods. These products can have up to 45 per cent trans fats. More and more are being used in French fries and other foods with labels claiming that they have been prepared with canola oil, without mentioning that the canola oil has first been hardened and is contributing trans fats. Health-conscious consumers often choose such products, believing them to be superior. Better labelling seems imperative to help people who would prefer to avoid trans fats. Until we get it, home-cooked chips fried in olive oil would be the healthiest choice.

In the United States, hydrogenated soy bean oil used in baking and frying has 30 to 50 per cent trans fatty acids. Margarines may have 23 per cent trans fats. The average intake of trans fatty acids in the United States is estimated to be 8 to 10 grams, although some researchers cite a range of intake from 1.6 to 38.7 grams a day. In the Netherlands, where fish and vegetable oils are commonly hydrogenated, daily consumption is estimated as 17 grams.

In Australia, researchers theorised that the daily intake of trans fatty acids would be much less. They based this on simulations of a typical diet and assumed that the major fats used in commercial foods were palm oil and beef tallow. Palm oil has no trans fatty acids and tallow has only low levels. With an increasing number of foods being prepared with hardened canola and soy bean oils, however, the level could go much higher. The actual intake by those people who eat more processed and prepared food would also be significantly higher than the assumed average levels. The significance of adverse effects of any particular food can be lost by averaging widely differing intakes. In a heterogenous population, some people eat a lot of processed and fatty foods; others eat none. Those on a high intake would do well to avoid foods processed with partially hydrogenated fats high in trans fatty acids.

Some fast food restaurants, upset at criticisms of their widespread use of saturated fats for frying, have opted for hydrogenated oil—a case of jumping out of the frying pan into the fire.

## FATS IN FOODS

Foods contain a mixture of types of fats, but particular foods are usually described by the dominant type of fatty acid. For example, olive oil is described as 'monounsaturated' because the major portion (about 72 per cent) of its fat is in the form of oleic acid, a monounsaturated fatty acid with 18 carbon atoms. Olive oil, however, also contains some saturated and some polyunsaturated fatty acids. When it is converted into an olive oil-based margarine, it may also gain some trans fatty acids as a result of the processing.

The dominant type of fatty acid present in a fat influences the melting point. The *cis* configuration in unsaturated fats causes bends or kinks, which makes it difficult for the carbon chains of fatty acids to join together and lowers their melting point. Saturated or trans fats have a higher melting point because their carbon atoms occur close together in a straight line, in crystalline structures that do not melt easily.

In the kitchen, you can get a good idea of which fatty acids predominate in foods by the solidity of the fat. Butter goes hard in the refrigerator because it has a high content of saturated fat. Adding some oil, as in dairy blend products, softens it because there is more unsaturated fat present. Beef fat is solid with its high percentage of saturated fatty acids and lamb fat is so saturated that it will harden in the griller at room temperature while you are eating your chops. Chicken and pork fat, by contrast, stay fairly soft even in the refrigerator. The fat in ocean trout or salmon is always soft because it is unsaturated. Most fish have this kind of fat so they won't freeze in their cold-water environment. Oils are liquid because of their high content of unsaturated fatty acids. The following table indicates the quantity of saturated, monounsaturated and polyunsaturated fat present in common foods.

| Food | Type of fat | | |
| --- | --- | --- | --- |
| | Saturated<br>g | Mono-<br>unsaturated<br>g | Poly-<br>unsaturated<br>g |
| *Oils* | | | |
| Canola oil, 100g | 7 | 63 | 30 |
| Coconut oil, 100g | 92 | 6 | 2 |
| Corn or maize oil, 100g | 14 | 32 | 54 |
| Cottonseed oil, 100g | 26 | 16 | 58 |
| Olive oil, 100g | 12 | 76 | 12 |
| Linseed oil,* 100g | 10 | 21 | 69* |
| Mono sun oil, ** 100g | 9 | 80 | 11 |
| Palm oil, 100g | 51 | 39 | 10 |
| Palm kernel oil, 100g | 84 | 14 | 2 |
| Peanut oil, 100g | 19 | 46 | 35 |
| Rice bran oil, 100g | 19 | 44 | 37 |
| Safflower oil, 100g | 10 | 14 | 76 |
| Soy bean oil, 100g | 15 | 23 | 62 |
| Sunflower oil, 100g | 11 | 23 | 66 |
| Sunola oil, *** 100g | 7 | 85 | 8 |
| *Other fats* | | | |
| Butter, 100g | 54 | 20 | 3 |

| Food | Type of fat | | |
| --- | --- | --- | --- |
| | Saturated g | Mono-unsaturated g | Poly-unsaturated g |
| Dairy blend spread, 100g | 42 | 23 | 15 |
| Dairy blend, reduced fat, 100g | 27 | 17 | 16 |
| Margarine, regular, 100g | 25 | 21 | 28 |
| Margarine, cooking, 100g | 38 | 36 | 6 |
| Margarine, polyunsaturated, 100g | 16 | 26** | 38 |
| Margarine, mono-unsaturated, 100g | 12 | 42** | 18 |
| Margarine spread, sunola, 100g | 12 | 39 | 9 |
| Lard, 100g | 40 | 45 | 15 |
| Beef dripping, 100g | 51 | 42 | 7 |
| Chicken fat, 100g | 31 | 48 | 21 |
| Copha, 100g | 98 | 2 | 0 |
| Chocolate, 100g | 61 | 36 | 3 |
| Mayonnaise, 1 tablespoon | 2 | 11 | 2 |
| *Nuts* | | | |
| Almonds, 100g | 5 | 34 | 14 |
| Brazil nuts, 100g | 16 | 26 | 23 |
| Cashew nuts, 100g | 9 | 28 | 9 |
| Chestnuts, 100g | 0 | 1 | 1 |
| Coconut, fresh, 100g | 31 | 2 | 1 |

| Food | Type of fat | | |
| --- | --- | --- | --- |
| | Saturated | Mono-unsaturated | Poly-unsaturated |
| | g | g | g |
| Coconut, desiccated, 100g | 53 | 4 | 2 |
| Coconut, creamed, block, 100g | 59 | 4 | 2 |
| Coconut cream, canned, 100g | 30g | 2 | 1 |
| Hazelnuts, 100g | 5 | 50 | 6 |
| Macadamia nuts, 100g | 11 | 61 | 2 |
| Peanuts, 100g | 8 | 21 | 14 |
| Peanut butter, 1 tablespoon | 2 | 5 | 3 |
| Pecans, 100g | 6 | 43 | 19 |
| Pine nuts, 100g | 5 | 20 | 41 |
| Pistachio nuts, weighed in the shell, 100g | 4 | 15 | 10 |
| Pumpkin seeds, 100g | 7 | 11 | 18 |
| Sesame seeds, 100g | 8 | 22 | 26 |
| Sunflower seeds, 100g | 4 | 10 | 31 |
| Tahini paste, 1 tablespoon | 2 | 4 | 5 |
| Walnuts, 100g | 6 | 12 | 48 |
| *Dairy products* | | | |
| Milk, 250 mL | 6 | 3 | 0 |
| Milk, fat-reduced, 250 mL | 2 | 1 | 0 |

| Food | Type of fat | | |
|------|-------------|---|---|
| | Saturated | Mono-unsaturated | Poly-unsaturated |
| | g | g | g |
| Cream, 2 tablespoons | 10 | 5 | 0 |
| Milk, goat's, 250 mL | 6 | 2 | 0 |
| Milk, sheep's, 250 mL | 10 | 4 | 1 |
| Soy beverage, 250 mL | 1 | 1 | 3 |
| Cheese, brie, 50g | 8 | 4 | 0 |
| Cheese, cheddar, 50g | 11 | 5 | 1 |
| Cheese, cottage, 100g | 2 | 1 | 0 |
| Cheese, cream, 50g | 15 | 7 | 1 |
| Cheese, feta, 50g | 7 | 2 | 0 |
| Cheese, mozzarella, 50g | 7 | 3 | 0 |
| Cheese, parmesan, 1 tablespoon | 3 | 1 | 0 |
| Cheese, ricotta, 50g | 3 | 1 | 0 |
| Yoghurt, natural, 200g | 3 | 2 | 0 |
| Ice-cream, 2 small scoops, 50g | 3 | 1 | 0 |
| *Other foods* | | | |
| Egg, 1 | 2 | 2 | 1 |
| Fish, grilled, 150g | 0.5 | 0.5 | 1 |
| Fish, orange roughy, grilled, 150g | 0.5 | 9 | 0 |

| Food | Type of fat | | |
| --- | --- | --- | --- |
| | Saturated g | Mono- unsaturated g | Poly- unsaturated g |
| Fish, salmon, grilled, 150g | 3 | 7 | 5 |
| Tuna, grilled, 150g | 1.5 | 1.5 | 2 |
| Prawns, 200g (weighed in the shell) | 0 | 0 | 0 |
| Octopus, 150g | 0.5 | 0.5 | 1 |
| Oysters, 12 | 0 | 0.5 | 0.5 |
| Salmon, canned, 100g | 2 | 4 | 2 |
| Beef, rump, grilled, lean, 150g | 3 | 3.5 | 0.5 |
| Lamb, grilled, lean, 150g | 5 | 3.5 | 1.5 |
| Pork steak, cooked, 150g | 3 | 3 | 1 |
| Chicken, roast, lean, 150g | 1.5 | 2.5 | 0.5 |
| Avocado, 100g | 4 | 12 | 2 |

\*  Linseed oil, also called flaxseed oil, has 54g/100g of alpha-linolenic acid, an
   omega 3 polyunsaturated fatty acid.
\*\*  These oils have been made from sunflowers bred to contain
   monounsaturated fat instead of their usual polyunsaturated fats.
\*\*\*  The monounsaturated fat in these products may be partly comprised of
   trans fats which may make up 12 to 15 per cent of the total fat content.

Some people are surprised to find that polyunsaturated and monounsaturated margarines

are a major source of saturated fats. The oils from which they are made usually contain quite low contents of saturated fatty acids. To turn these oils into more spreadable products, they are combined with fats high in saturated or trans fatty acids. Some have a bit of both. If margarines did not have some saturated or trans fats, they would still be oils. In making poly and mono-unsaturated margarines, unsaturated oils are combined with enough saturated fats or trans fatty acids to form a spread. It is not possible to have a spreadable fat without one or other of these less desirable components. Even if the major type of fat present is unsaturated, margarines, like butter, consist of 80 per cent fat, so the number of grams of saturated fat in an average serving is high. For example, a tablespoon of poly or mono-unsaturated margarine has almost a teaspoon of saturated and trans fat (as well as its other fats) whereas the much-maligned egg has less than half a teaspoon of saturated fat. Many people avoid eggs but happily use margarine on toast, in mashed potato, for frying and in cooking. Most have the mistaken idea that unsaturated mar-garines do not contain any saturated fat.

Chocolate and beef fat are both high in the saturated fatty acid stearic acid. This does not increase blood levels of LDL cholesterol, a point often made by confectionery manufacturers. There are several other facts that are important, however. Chocolate is also rich in palmitic acid which *does* raise LDL cholesterol levels. Stearic acid also increases the tendency of blood to form clots. An analysis of chocolate reveals that many chocolates contain little cocoa butter and a lot of palm and palm kernel oil. Sadly for chocolate lovers, there is little that can be said in favour of the fats in chocolate, except that they taste appealing to most people.

## PERCENTAGE ENERGY FROM FAT

Some people prefer to consider the percentage of kilojoules that come from fat rather than thinking in terms of grams of fat. For example, health authorities are aiming to reduce Australians' average fat consumption from about 40 per cent of energy to less than 30 per cent. Some people wish to be very strict and reduce fat to no more than 10 per cent of their kilojoules.

When we have a complete list of someone's food intake for the day, we can calculate the number of grams of protein, fat, carbohydrate and alcohol, and then work out what percentage of the energy comes from each. This method is less appropriate to work out an ideal energy percentage for any particular food and almost impossible for the average person to calculate each day.

One hundred per cent of the energy in all foods must come from protein, fat or carbohydrate. Foods that do not contain carbohydrate, such as meat or fish, must therefore derive all their kilojoules from protein and fat. For example, a 150 g piece of fish may have 2 grams of fat and 20 grams of protein. The 2 grams of fat provide 74 kJ of energy and the protein provides 340 kJ. The total kilojoule level for the piece of fish is 414 kJ, of which fat provides 18 per cent. Those who want a very low fat diet may therefore reject such fish, even though the absolute amount of fat is very low.

Another example can be seen in the absurdity of people who won't add a slurp of milk to their tea because milk has 52 per cent of its kilojoules coming from fat. The actual fat content of a slurp of milk in a cup of tea or coffee is about half a gram, which is negligible.

It makes much more sense for people concerned about controlling or losing body fat to aim for a particular number of grams of fat each day. For those needing to lose weight, an intake of 30 to 40 grams would be appropriate.

# THE RANCIDITY AND OXIDATION OF FATS

Fats become rancid, or go 'off', when oxygen attacks their fatty acid chain in a process known as oxidation. Some types of fatty acids oxidise or go 'off' more rapidly than others. Omega 3 fatty acids, such as those found in linseed oil or fish, are the least stable and the most likely to oxidise if exposed to oxygen in the air. That is why fish does not keep long and why fish that isn't fresh can be picked by its aroma. It is also a major reason why it is difficult to enjoy the benefits of linseed oil.

Canola oil also contains some omega 3 fatty acids that oxidise easily. If you have ever tried deep-frying with canola, or even shallow-frying for more than a minute or two, you may have noticed a fishy smell. It comes from the break-down of the omega 3 fatty acid: alpha-linolenic acid.

The richest source of alpha-linolenic acid is linseed (or flax) oil. It is so unstable that it can be kept only for a short time, and then only if it is cold and in a brown bottle away from light. Once attacked by oxygen, the breakdown of its fatty acids is inevitable. For this reason it is difficult to use it for cooking. Keeping linseeds inside their protective coating in a cool place is the best way to prevent the fats from becoming rancid. Australians generally do not consume linseed oil but rub it into cricket bats or add it to paints, for which it is excellent because the oxidation process means it will dry quickly. Linseeds themselves are becoming more popular and are now added to some breads.

Omega 6 fatty acids found in polyunsaturated

oils also oxidise readily during storage and cooking, and also in cell membranes in the body. A single use in deep-frying breaks down some of the fats in polyunsaturated oils through a process known as hydro-peroxidation. The compounds formed then destroy the oil's anti-oxidants so that it then oxidises rapidly. Polyunsaturated oils should only ever be used once. Any leftovers after frying should be thrown out. Olive oil, by contrast, has such high levels of naturally occurring anti-oxidants as well as mainly monounsaturated fat that it can be used many times before any undesirable fatty acids form. In practice this more than compensates for its initial high price.

Once polyunsaturated fats take up residence in cell membranes or as part of low-density lipoproteins in arteries, the requirement for antioxidants also increases. The recommended daily intake of vitamin E, one of the anti-oxidant vitamins, is thus directly related to the intake of polyunsaturated fatty acids. Some of these fats are also good sources of vitamin E but this may be destroyed by cooking or some types of processing. Most commercial oils are extracted using a chemical solvent, which must then be removed, but this means that many of the original protective substances are also removed. Again, olive oil has an advantage as it is produced by cold pressing. Only olive oil marked 'pomace oil' is extracted with a chemical solvent.

Very short-chain saturated fatty acids found in butter and dairy products also oxidise easily and give rise to the slightly 'off' flavour in butter that is no longer fresh. The fats from goats' and sheep milk also oxidise readily and this is presented as a 'plus' because it contributes to the distinctive flavour of the cheeses made from these milks.

The oxidation of fats is commonly called rancidity. It is undesirable from a gastronomic viewpoint and also harmful for health because oxidised fatty acids can damage arteries. Anti-oxidants help prevent oxidation. Most margarines and some oils and cooking fats have an anti-oxidant added to prevent rancidity, as many of their natural anti-oxidants are destroyed by processing.

Makers of processed and fast foods use vegetable oils that have been converted into saturated fats or trans fatty acids because they are less likely to oxidise and therefore have a longer shelf life than that of the unsaturated oils from which they are made.

# CHAPTER 3

# Some health advantages and disadvantages of fats

Until recently, most people throughout the world considered fat was good. In the quantities that many ate, it probably was. There is now a common misconception spreading throughout the developed world that fat is undesirable, but the effects of fat on health depend primarily on the quantity and type of fats consumed. Some fatty acids are essential at all ages, a certain amount of fat is important, and it is vital for growth and survival during infancy. In most Western countries, however, the intake of *saturated* fats has become excessive and is related to many health problems.

## FAT IN THE DIET OF INFANTS

Infants have a greater need for fat than any other age group. For the first few days of life a newborn baby gets colostrum from its mother's breasts. Colostrum is high in protein and rich in compounds that give the baby immunity to infection. There is less fat in colostrum than in mature breast milk, but more than twice as much cholesterol.

Colostrum is also rich in fat-soluble vitamins—about three times the level present in mature breast milk. At all ages, fat-soluble vitamins need dietary fat for their absorption.

As the colostrum gives way to transitional milk, the fat content rises and the cholesterol falls slightly. When mature milk comes in on about the third or fourth day, it has even more fat. The breastfed infant continues to get more than half its kilojoules from fat and this level is vitally important to provide the baby with a package of concentrated energy for fast growth. Ideally, breastfeeding should continue for the baby's first 12 months, with solid foods commencing when the baby is about 6 months old. For the first year, the high fat content and other important nutrients of milk play a major role in the infant's growth.

Infant formulas also have a high content of fat, although the types of fatty acids cannot match those of breast milk. Most infant formulas are made from cow's milk, with additional vegetable fats to try to make them resemble breast milk more closely. The fatty acids in cow's milk are so different from those in breast milk, however, that even an infant formula that contains essential fatty acids still does not achieve a similar profile of fatty acids.

In breast milk, saturated fats predominate and its cholesterol content is still slightly higher than that of cow's milk. There is also a relatively high

## Major percentages of fatty acids in human milk, cow's milk and average infant formula

| Fatty acid | Human milk | Cow's milk | Modified infant formula* |
|---|---|---|---|
| **Saturated fat (total %)** | 46 | 67 | 43 |
| Butyric C4:0 | 0 | 3.2 | 0 |
| Caproic C6:0 | 0 | 2.0 | 0.1 |
| Caprylic C8:0 | 0 | 1.2 | 1.6 |
| Capric C10:0 | 1.4 | 2.8 | 1.2 |
| Lauric C12:0 | 5.4 | 3.5 | 9.3 |
| Myristic C14:0 | 7.3 | 11.2 | 4.1 |
| Palmitic C16:0 | 26.5 | 26.0 | 22.0 |
| Stearic C18:0 | 9.5 | 11.2 | 4.3 |
| **Monounsaturated (total %)** | 41 | 30 | 38 |
| Palmitoleic C16:1 | 4.0 | 2.7 | 0.1 |
| Oleic C18:1 | 35.4 | 27.8 | 38.0 |
| Gadoleic C20:1 | 0.5 | 0 | 0 |
| **Polyunsaturated (total %)** | 13 | 3 | 19 |
| Linoleic C18:2 n–6 | 9** | 1.4 | 17.2 |
| Alpha-linolenic C18:3 n–3 | 0.8 | 1.5 | 1.8 |
| Docosahexaenoic acid DHA C22:6 n–3 | 0.2 | 0 | 0 |

\*    Infant formula milks differ. These figures are taken from brands designed to
     resemble human breast milk as closely as possible.

\*\*   Varies according to mother's diet. Those who consume more linoleic acid
     have greater quantities in their breast milk.

level of polyunsaturated omega 3 fatty acids, especially docosahexaenoic acid, or DHA. Infant formula milks do not contain these very long-chain fatty acids, although many now add alpha-linolenic acid as well as high quantities of linoleic acid. The formula-fed infant must then convert these fatty acids into the essential longer-chain fatty acids. The breastfed infant gets these fatty acids supplied ready-made. Supplements of DHA to add to formula milks will help to some extent.

Initial research into omega 3 fatty acids concentrated on eicosapentaenoic acid or EPA, a high quantity of which occurs in fish, especially those living in very cold waters. Because EPA is strongly related to lower levels of blood clots and coronary heart disease, it was considered the most important omega 3 fatty acid. Others, such as DHA, were largely ignored and even considered inferior. Some medical researchers were quite dispirited when they found that most Australian fish from the warmer waters of the Great Barrier Reef had more DHA and less EPA. Others dismissed the importance of EPA because it was present only in very small quantities in breast milk.

It was not until some researchers realised that breast milk contained high levels of DHA and began to look for a role for this fatty acid that it gained status, eventually overtaking EPA in this respect. We still do not know everything about omega 3 fatty acids in breast milk, but we do know that DHA goes into the retina of the baby's eye and into the brain. It is not possible to research its effects on the brain, but studies show that breastfed babies have sharper vision than those fed on formula milks, probably for at least their first 6 months. DHA also goes into red blood cells and over the next few years we will almost certainly discover other benefits.

There are claims that children who were breastfed as babies have higher intelligence quotients (IQ) than other children. Researchers who have come up with statistics to prove this have tried to account for the fact that mothers who breastfeed have higher education levels, but it is almost impossible to isolate such factors. Claims about breast milk fatty acids and IQ must therefore be regarded as unproven.

There is no generally accepted theory about why so much of the fat in breast milk is saturated or why its cholesterol level is so high. Some researchers have suggested that when the diet provides ready-made cholesterol, the infant's liver will no longer need to make its own supplies and will be more able to turn off its cholesterol-synthesis mechanism when it is not needed in later life. Others think it is simply that infants need high levels of cholesterol to produce plenty of the bile acids required for emulsifying the high-fat diet that is essential for their rapid growth.

The triglycerides in breast milk are also interesting in that the 2-position on the glycerol backbone is always occupied by either myristic or palmitic acids—saturated fatty acids that increase blood cholesterol levels. These, too, may be needed to support growth.

The pattern of fatty acids in breast milk should be a guide for manufacturers of infant formulas. Most aim to match the natural product and many have been trying to find a way to introduce more omega 3 fatty acids into infant formulas. They cannot simply add DHA because it is an unstable molecule and oxidises readily to form harmful compounds. Alpha-linolenic acid, a potential building block for DHA, is also unstable, but some manufacturers have overcome technical difficulties and incorporated it into some of their products.

A few years ago there were claims that formula milks were superior to human milk because they had more polyunsaturated fatty acids and less cholesterol. This is the sort of crazy thinking that comes from researchers concentrating on a single aspect of human nutrition for one group only, then applying it to another. Unsaturated fats and low levels of dietary cholesterol may be important for the middle-aged male or older woman at high risk of coronary heart disease, but such issues are not relevant to growing infants.

## FAT IN THE DIET OF CHILDREN

Whatever type of milk they are being given, all infants need enough fat to provide sufficient kilojoules for growth. Once they are eating a wider variety of foods, children still need a milk that provides fat. They also need a source of vitamin A. Low-fat milk does not provide this vitamin. Adults can convert beta-carotene in fruits and vegetables into vitamin A but children do not do this efficiently for several years. The fat in milk is also important for the absorption of vitamins A, D, E and K. Children should therefore have regular milk, at least for their first few years. There is no problem in using low-fat milk in custards or other occasional foods.

As in infancy, children do not need lots of obviously fatty foods with poor nutrient levels. Instead, they should get their fat from products such as eggs, lean meat or poultry, cereals, avocado, peanut (or other nut) butter, milk, cheese and yoghurt, all of which supply nutrients important for growth and activity. A scrape of butter or margarine on toast fingers is unlikely to cause problems, although it is not necessary.

High-fat extras such as crisps, chocolate, biscuits, cakes, pastries and fast foods have no essential purpose and should be omitted or used only as occasional extras. Many people do not see any problem with children eating a lot of these junk foods with high levels of fat, assuming that children are active enough to burn them up. They ignore the dental hazards of sweet fatty foods such as biscuits, cakes and confectionery.

In days gone by, when children walked long distances and helped with heavy household tasks, some junk foods may not have been such a problem. Somewhat ironically, few such foods were available then. These days, however, about one quarter of school-aged children in countries such as Australia, Canada, the United States and Singapore are overweight. The problem of child obesity is also increasing in Japan and other countries that are increasing their consumption of fatty junk foods.

There is no doubt that part of the blame for excess weight lies with decreasing physical activity that comes from children playing computer games and watching videos instead of playing outside, being driven to school instead of walking, and having few energy-consuming household tasks allotted to them. But some blame for the high level of excess weight in children must also go to the food they eat. Where once children ate bread, they now eat biscuits; instead of fruit, they are more likely to eat crisps and other fatty snack foods; and chocolates, biscuits, takeaway foods and other fried items that were once reserved for special occasions have now become everyday fare. A diet high in such fatty foods can easily lead to excess weight. This subject is discussed further in chapter 4.

# THE DISADVANTAGES OF FATS

The advantages of fats have been listed in chapter 1. There are also major disadvantages. These include the role of fat in excess weight and obesity, mature onset diabetes (also called non-insulin dependent diabetes mellitus or NIDDM), coronary heart disease, high blood pressure, gallstones and certain types of cancer, especially of the bowel, prostate and endometrium. The influence of dietary fat on obesity is discussed in greater detail in chapter 4.

All types of fat are involved in excess weight. Not all fats, however, can be criticised for other health problems. Some fats are worse than others and some may have benefits. Contrary to popular belief, we should not categorise fats as good or bad depending on whether they come from vegetable or animal sources. Some of the worst fats are of vegetable origin and some of the most useful occur in fish. The important point is not to damn all fats, which is sometimes done by those whose main aim is to promote ultra slenderness. Some fats have a long and distinguished role in the diet and we avoid them at our peril.

## SATURATED FATS AND CORONARY HEART DISEASE

High levels of saturated fats in the diets of adults almost certainly deserve some condemnation for their role in various types of heart disease. Until the 1950s, most nutrition researchers thought the key to good health was to have plenty of food, especially foods rich in animal protein. This was an understandable viewpoint, as up to that time most nutrition-related health problems were due to a lack of some nutrient, or a general lack of food. Those in countries blessed with a rich supply of food, including high-fat meats and dairy products, appeared to have few problems, except among the poor who could not afford enough to eat.

During the 1950s, coronary heart disease reached almost epidemic proportions in wealthy countries, especially among middle-aged men. Researchers began to look for reasons. They soon discovered the link with cigarette smoking, and by the 1960s and 1970s began to direct anti-smoking campaigns at men. As a result, many men gave up smoking and, by the 1980s, the heart disease rate dropped. With blue-collar workers anti-smoking campaigns were less successful and heart disease rates did not fall.

## Research into saturated fats

In the 1950s a group of researchers led by Dr Ancel Keys coordinated a now famous study known as the Seven Countries Study in which they looked at deaths from coronary heart disease and dietary patterns in eighteen populations in seven different countries. This study is still continuing and has given rise to many others.

Keys and his co-workers found that the total *amount* of fat that people ate had no relationship to coronary heart disease, but the *type* of fat was highly relevant. People in countries such as Greece ate the most fat but had the least heart disease. Almost all the fat came from olive oil and nuts, with some from cheese and yoghurt. Mediterranean populations were not vegetarian but they ate little meat, and cakes, pastries and other such goodies were eaten only for feasts and special occasions. Vegetables made palatable with herbs, garlic, lemon and olive oil featured strongly in their diets, along with fish, bread, other grain products and a moderate, regular intake of red wine.

At the other end of the spectrum, people in Finland had the highest rate of heart disease. They also ate a lot of fat but it came mainly from meat, butter, milk and processed fats. Their vegetable consumption was low and they drank little red wine.

The total amount of fat consumed did not significantly differ between the diets of Finland and Greece, but the types of fats did. The Finnish diet, and that of populations with similarly high levels of heart disease, were dominated by saturated fat. These fats had only a minor role in the diet of all countries with low rates of heart disease.

The Japanese populations studied also had low levels of coronary heart disease, but high levels of high blood pressure and stroke. Their diet was low in all fats, including saturated fats. Vegetables, fish and rice were dominant foods. Their salt intake from soy sauce and salted fish was high and directly related to blood pressure and stroke.

## The move to polyunsaturated fats

In spite of the importance and great publicity given to the Seven Countries Study, one of their essential findings was overlooked for many years. You might think that researchers would have gone back to the United States and told them to eat like the Greeks or the Southern Italians. But in their rush to condemn saturated fats such as butter and find an alternative, researchers and the food industry ignored the types of fats, and other foods, that Mediterranean people were eating.

To some extent, this ignorance had a political basis. Few dietary changes are free of bias and most recommendations are pushed by someone who stands to make a profit from them. In this case, the oilseed industry saw a splendid opportunity to introduce a new range of highly profitable products—polyunsaturated oils and margarines.

Advertisers made the most of the research findings that saturated fats were undesirable and that an alternative to a highly saturated product such as butter was highly preferable. They vigorously promoted polyunsaturated margarines along with safflower, sunflower, corn and soy bean oils, and health authorities supported these products at the time.

Research studies were carried out to support these assumptions, but these had an artificiality that distorted the results. Subjects were given experimental liquid diets containing different types of fats, and their blood cholesterol levels were measured. When these diets contained a lot of saturated fats, cholesterol levels rose. With large quantities of polyunsaturated fats, the levels fell. When given monounsaturated fats, similar to those found in olive oil, their blood cholesterol levels did not change significantly. At this stage saturated fats were damned, polyunsaturated fats were praised and mono-unsaturates were largely ignored. Researchers overlooked the observation that people in Mediterranean countries who ate large quantities of monounsaturated fats in the form of olive oil had low blood cholesterol levels, and at the time the lowest rate of coronary heart disease in the world. For the next 30 years researchers and health authorities concentrated on polyunsaturated fats and referred to P:S ratios (polyunsaturated to saturated), and in some quarters this tendency persists even now. They ignored monounsaturated fats, even though they make up the bulk of fatty acids in many diets. It is not clear that the P:S ratio ever did more than simply indicate the quantity of polyunsaturated oils and margarine being consumed, but the ratio is still quoted. Its continued appeal demonstrates how usage tends to create status which persists long after usefulness has ended.

More than 30 years ago some researchers also showed that different saturated fatty acids did not have equal effects in raising serum cholesterol. The confectionery industry picked up the fact that stearic acid, a saturated fatty acid that does *not* raise cholesterol, was present in chocolate. They did not give equal publicity to the fact that chocolate is also high in palmitic acid, which *does* raise blood cholesterol. Nor did they publicise the fact that stearic acid may cause blood platelets to stick together, increasing the chances of blood clots forming. This is an example of how research into fatty acids can be used to suit the purposes of a particular group with a product to sell.

In practice, most foods that are high in saturated fat contain a mixture of these fats rather than just one, and cutting back on all foods rich in saturated fats is the easiest way to reduce the less desirable saturated fatty acids. I have mentioned it as an example of how messages about diet and heart disease can be oversimplified so that they convey something other than the full truth. Some researchers and health authorities seem keen to protect the public from facts that they (the authorities) deem to be too complicated for them (the public). Some researchers also become carried away with the results of test-tube meals and ignore the importance of the total diet.

## The move to monounsaturates

The advice to everyone to increase polyunsaturated fats was strange, especially in light of the fact that no human population had ever consumed such large quantities of these fats. Polyunsaturated fats started their fall from grace during the 1970s and 1980s when medical researchers realised the importance of distinguishing between LDL-cholesterol, which increases the risk of heart disease (the so-called 'bad' cholesterol), and HDL-cholesterol ('good' cholesterol), which reduces the risk. Once again, they examined the effects of different classes of dietary fats given to volunteers.

Saturated fats increased both types of blood cholesterol, although their effect on the 'good' HDL type was small compared with their effect in raising 'bad' LDL-cholesterol. Polyunsaturated fats, given in high quantity, turned out to lower both 'good' and 'bad' cholesterol levels—hence their assumed potency when only the total levels were being measured. Monounsaturated fats, on the other hand, lowered 'bad' cholesterol and seemed to have some potential to raise the 'good' type.

The conclusion at this stage was that saturated fats were still bad, and that polyunsaturates were undesirable in large doses but essential in small quantities. Researchers began to sing the praises of monounsaturated fats and manufacturers looked at ways of producing more of them.

The next stage in this saga of unfolding scientific research has occurred over the past 10 years. The 'bad' LDL-cholesterol turns out to be a true villain only when it oxidises. Polyunsaturated fats oxidise more readily than the more stable mono-unsaturates, mainly because the polyunsaturates have less stable double bonds in their molecules. This is why oils with a high content of polyunsaturated fat go rancid quickly in the kitchen. It occurs in the frying pan, especially if a polyunsaturated oil is used more than once. Oxidation can also occur in the arteries, where free radical molecules produced as body tissues age attack polyunsaturated fats carried in low-density lipoproteins. Once these fats are degraded by the oxidation reaction, they are taken up into foam cells and also form substances that increase the chances of blood cells clumping together to form a clot. Oxidised fats also lead to the formation of more inflammatory compounds, and interfere with the ability of the cells lining the artery to relax.

This oxidation reaction does not occur readily with saturated fatty acids and is slow with mono-unsaturated fatty acids. But a diet high in polyunsaturates can present a greater risk for atherosclerosis, unless more anti-oxidants are also supplied to prevent oxidation. In nature, most polyunsaturated fats occur with plenty of anti-oxidants. When they are refined, however, many of the protective accompaniments are lost.

It is worthwhile looking at the history of dietary recommendations for coronary heart disease because they illustrate how greater knowledge can alter the emphasis in dietary advice. The early studies emphasised the effects of diet on total serum cholesterol, until it became known that the sub-fraction of cholesterol that increases the risk of coronary heart disease is carried in low-density lipoproteins (LDL). Cholesterol in high-density lipoproteins (HDL) decreases the risk of coronary heart disease.

The change of emphasis does not invalidate the conclusions drawn from the initial studies. It just means that they did not look at the whole picture. The nature of the intricate work being done by most researchers means that many will continue to attach great importance to the single issue they are studying.

Some people will use any point disputed by nutritional scientists to justify not doing anything, although there does not seem to be too much confusion in their buying habits. When told that polyunsaturated margarine was good for them, people bought it. The fact that it was easily spreadable and cheaper than butter probably helped sales, but it was the health message that won people over to a product they had rejected, because of its taste, before the mid-1970s. Now that they are hearing health messages about monounsaturated fats, people are switching to monounsaturated margarine and buying and enjoying olive oil. Sales of olive oil have increased dramatically over the past couple of years—formerly, only small bottles of it were sold in pharmacies or the therapeutic goods section of the supermarket, but olive oil now dominates the oil section. Where confusion does arise, it could be due to conflicting sales pitches from those who are marketing foods rich in mono- or polyunsaturates.

Saturated fats are still damned—and there is no evidence to support reinstating them to any positive health status—but mono-unsaturates have at last been accepted. Unfortunately, some people have taken the anti-fat message to heart so much that they want to condemn all fats. This may not turn out to be wise.

When people eat very little fat of any kind, their blood levels of LDL-cholesterol are low. They produce very little LDL-cholesterol and their bodies break down very little. A moderate intake of saturated fats and a high intake of monounsaturated fats, as consumed in Mediterranean countries, produces intermediate levels of LDL-cholesterol and high breakdown rates. By contrast, a high intake of saturated fats and a low consumption of mono-unsaturates, as occurs in parts of Northern Europe, produces lots of LDL-cholesterol and very little is broken down.

LDL-cholesterol production is due to eating a lot of saturated fat. The breakdown of LDL-cholesterol is greater with a higher intake of monounsaturated fatty acids, so these fats may protect us against the damaging effects of high blood cholesterol. Polyunsaturates have a lesser role in this respect.

## Anti-oxidants

A new player entered the arena when theories about oxidation became accepted. Anti-oxidants are now big news—and selling well. As their name suggests, anti-oxidants can prevent oxidation reactions. Foods contain literally thousands of anti-oxidants: vegetables, fruits, nuts, olive oil, red wine and tea are the major sources. With the exception of tea, all these foods dominate the Mediterranean diets. We could probably have saved 40 years of going round in a circle if we had taken note of what Mediterranean people ate and followed suit. We might also have taken up some of the obvious pleasures that Mediterranean people enjoy as they sit down with friends and family to their wonderfully tasty and healthy foods. We should also learn from this that no single food is responsible for good health. Olive oil has mainly monounsaturated fats, which are now acknowledged as beneficial. But olive oil also contains dozens of potent anti-oxidants which may be equally beneficial. This point is still being ignored by those who produce and market other monounsaturated oils that lack olive oil's variety of anti-oxidants. There are advertisements carrying Mediterranean recipes that use highly processed canola oil, genetically engineered from rape seeds to remove their harmful erucic acid, extracted with a solvent and containing one added anti-oxidant to replace those lost during processing. This product may well be a useful oil, but it has nothing to do with the virtues of the Mediterranean diet. It reduces LDL-cholesterol levels nicely, but we simply do not know its other effects at this stage. Perhaps its worst feature is that it has been processed to have no flavour—just when we are learning that many of the most potent anti-oxidants are found in the flavour components of foods.

Once again, however, the research has been oversimplified and hampered by people trying to push particular products. Sales of anti-oxidant vitamins (A, C and E) are at an all-time high: the advertisements imply that they will save you from the effects of fat. Folate is also an anti-oxidant vitamin, but does not seem to be promoted on this basis to any extent. Perhaps its name is still unfamiliar to many people. Most of the most potent anti-oxidants in foods have even less familiar names, many of them difficult to pronounce, which will make it hard to market any of them as supplements. Such a move would also be absurd, as the fact that they exist in their thousands may well be the major reason for their potency.

Natural foods are amazingly complex mixtures of compounds, and a growing body of research is showing that many substances work quite differently when isolated from their companion compounds. This was shown in studies of beta-carotene and cancer. There are now over 200 studies showing that those who eat the most fruit and vegetables have the least cancer at almost every site in the body. The first assumption was that the vitamins in these foods were responsible. Four major long-term trials looking at the effects of beta-carotene on lung cancer and bowel polyps found that those given the vitamin had more lung cancer and polyps than those given the placebo pills. The original studies were not wrong in claiming protective effects from fruit and vegetables, but they wrongly assumed that the benefit came from vitamins. Fruit and vegetables contain several thousand different compounds.

## A selection of anti-oxidant-rich foods

| Food | Anti-oxidants present* |
|------|------------------------|
| Apples | bioflavonoids |
| Basil | O-cimene, cineol, esdragol |
| Broad beans | flavonoids (especially quercetin) |
| Broccoli & brassicas | carotenoids, plant sterols, dithiolthiones, glucosinolates (indoles), isothiocyanates |
| Capers | biflavones, resins, glucosides |
| Capsicum | capsaicin, carotenoids |
| Carrots | carotenoids, coumarins, flavonoids |
| Citrus fruits | carotenoids, flavonoids, limonoids, coumarins, monoterpenes, triterpenoids |
| Eggplant | phenols, plant sterols, saponins |
| Fennel | phenols, esdragol, anethole |
| Garlic | glucosides, allyl methyl trisulphide, allylic sulphides, allicin, γ-glutamyl, allylic cysteines |
| Ginger | curcumins, gingerols, diarylhptanoids |
| Horseradish | isothiocyanates |
| Linseeds | α linolenic acid, lignans |
| Marjoram | terpineol, borneol, rosmarinic acid |
| Mint | menthol, cineol, menthoruran, terpenes |
| Olives & olive oil | phenols |

| Food | Anti-oxidants present* |
|------|------------------------|
| Onions | flavonoids, many sulphur compounds |
| Oregano | thymol, terpenes, carnarole, ursolic acid |
| Parsley | coumarins, carotenoids (especially lutein), flavonoids, monoterpenes, phenols, phthalides, polyacetalenes, apiin, pinene |
| Purslane | α linolenic acid, carotenoids |
| Rosemary | pinene, borneol, carnosol, ursolic acid |
| Sage | borneol, camphor, cineol, tuyone, tannins, ursolic acid |
| Soy beans | phytoestrogens, flavonoids |
| Tea, green or black | tannins, including polyphenols, catechins |
| Thyme | thymol, terpenes, tannins, carnarole |
| Tomatoes (red, ripe) | carotenoids, especially lycopene, coumarins (especially quercetin), plant sterols |
| Vegetables | carotenoids, numerous anti-oxidants |
| Wine, red | polyphenols, including resveratrol |

## Which changes are best?

Over-simplified messages in advertisements and on food labels can lead to changes that are not necessarily ideal, and may at best be compromises. We must always look at why certain products are being promoted and whether promotions convey the full message. For example, plant geneticists have been busily changing sunflowers to decrease their usual polyunsaturated fatty acids and to increase their monounsaturate content. This is to give a more marketable ingredient for margarine now that there is widespread criticism of high intakes of polyunsaturated products. But is it necessary, or would it be better to eat some regular sunflower seeds and skip margarine altogether? Some polyunsaturated fatty acids are essential to the diet. Sunflower seeds have always been a well-balanced source, supplying plenty of anti-oxidants along with their polyunsaturated fatty acids. Will these still be present in the same proportions once the fatty acids are changed in the genetically modified monounsaturated sunflowers? The plant, after all, produces its anti-oxidants to match the needs of its fats.

At other times, too, a little knowledge has been a dangerous thing. Linseeds are a valuable source of alpha-linolenic acid, an omega 3 fatty acid. In fact, linseeds are so rich in this highly unstable fatty acid that the oil goes rancid within hours or days of being squeezed from the seeds. (The short lifespan of its fatty acids is one reason why linseed oil is used in paints and to rub on cricket bats.) Some researchers decided linseed oil could be used as a food if the plants were engineered so that they had less of this easily oxidised fatty acid. The oil extracted from the new plant was christened linola. Since then, however, we have discovered omega 3 fatty acids are the valuable part of linseeds. The new highly polyunsaturated linola oil took a wrong turning, thanks to the incomplete knowledge of the time. Eating linseeds themselves solves some of the problems of oxidation. As long as they are kept in the fridge, the oil is protected within the seeds. Food manufacturers, however, see linseeds as much less attractive, since few people will consume such great quantities as they might with a margarine made from their oil. This is where commercial food interests and good nutrition are incompatible. Wise eating demands moderation; marketing wants ever-increasing consumption.

## CHOLESTEROL

The message that *cholesterol is harmful* is another example of a simple message that went wrong. Most people are unaware of distinctions between the cholesterol in foods and blood cholesterol. One does not necessarily lead to another, and concentrating on food sources of cholesterol has led to some inappropriate changes and neglect of the real problem. For example, most Australians who are told they have high blood cholesterol cut out eggs. This is a simple response to a simple message and is very common, but since eggs contribute less than 2 per cent of the fat in the Australian diet, the message may be inappropriate.

The fact that most people now believe that eggs are bad for them and have therefore stopped eating them may also result in undesirable dietary changes. Since eggs are not a major source of saturated fat in the diet, and since foods eaten as substitutes may have high levels of saturated fat, the over-simplified message may produce the wrong effect. For example, an egg has 5.2 grams of total fat and less than 2 grams of saturated fat. If it is replaced by a bowl of toasted muesli with fat-reduced milk (which most people think is a healthy choice), the fat content in the new 'healthier' choice will amount to 10 grams of total fat, carrying 5 grams of saturated fat.

We must also question whether certain community groups may be disadvantaged by removing eggs from their diet. The *real* message to reduce blood cholesterol is to cut back on saturated fat. The once standard breakfast of fatty fried bacon and fried eggs was high in fat and saturated fat, but its demise has turned an entire population off a nutritious food, which can also be easily incorporated into many low-fat, inexpensive meals. When many people wanted a quick, easy meal, and would have once used eggs, they now have fast foods, most of which have a much higher content of fat. Two eggs on toast has less than half the fat of a fast food hamburger.

The desire for a simple message—*cholesterol is bad*—has led to confusion between dietary and blood cholesterol. A more complicated message might have conveyed a more accurate message.

Could the public have coped with it? Health authorities and the food industry assumed they could not. As a result we may have failed to achieve the most appropriate dietary change.

## REPLACING SATURATED FATS

In France, Spain, Greece and Southern Italy, people eat large quantities of cheese and yoghurt, yet rates of coronary heart disease are low. It may be that other foods such as vegetables, olive oil, nuts and red wine provide enough protection against the undesirable properties of the saturated fats in cheese and yoghurt. It is also possible that when milk is fermented to make cheese and yoghurt, alterations in either the arrangement of fatty acids on their triglyceride backbone or some aspect of the changes in proteins in the foods overrides the saturated fats. We simply do not know the answer at this stage. But such strong evidence does make us consider whether it is good to advise people to remove as much saturated fat as possible from the diet. Perhaps we only need to reduce the excessive saturated fat that can dominate the diet from fast foods, foods fried in saturated animal or vegetable fats, biscuits, pastries, butter, cream, margarine and confectionery.

The two most likely contenders to replace excess saturated fat are starchy foods or monounsaturated fats. There are historical precedents and evidence supporting both courses of action.

The healthy diet that contributes to longevity in Japan has lots of rice to provide kilojoules from its starchy carbohydrate, as well as vegetables, legumes, some nuts, fish and other seafoods, and fresh fruit. Other foods have traditionally been used only in small quantities.

The healthy Mediterranean diets use mono-unsaturated fats as a major source of kilojoules. They come mostly from olive oil, with nuts also an important source, along with other commonly consumed foods rich in protective anti-oxidants.

The debate about which is the best substitute for excess saturated fat is likely to go on for some time. Meanwhile, the traditional diets that have proved protective against coronary heart disease are disappearing in their places of origin as fast food companies and food manufacturers move in to increase their world market dominance, and as local people adopt American-style eating habits for convenience in their increasingly time-strapped lives. As a result, we are already seeing increases in coronary heart disease and decreases in longevity in countries such as Greece, and similar effects are expected in Japan as risk factors increase with changing ways of life.

In Lyon, France, people who had already had one heart attack were randomly assigned either to a Mediterranean-style diet or one based on low-fat recommendations from the American Heart Association. Blood cholesterol levels stayed much the same in each group but there was a 70 per cent reduction in deaths from heart attacks in the group given the Mediterranean diet. This dramatic reduction occurred without any significant reduction in blood cholesterol.

The only similar trials that have successfully reduced deaths from heart attacks and other coronary events were conducted in Wales where an increased fish intake was given credit, and a Norwegian trial in which participants reduced saturated fat without increasing polyunsaturated fat and ate more fish, fruit and vegetables.

These trials are important because none of them used a diet high in the kind of polyunsaturated fats that heart associations have recommended since the 1950s, even though no intervention/prevention trial has ever found it successful in preventing coronary deaths.

A diet high in the kind of polyunsaturates found in margarine and many vegetable oils (linoleic acid) does reduce blood cholesterol and there is no doubt that this is important. But lowering total blood cholesterol is only one factor, and by itself may not always be enough to decrease deaths from coronary heart disease and other causes.

The chief researcher in the Lyon study has shown that when linoleic acid is increased enough to reduce blood cholesterol, blood platelets may stick together more, increasing the risk of blood clots forming. Eating more fish will help prevent this.

The authors of the Lyon Diet Heart Study suggest that the protective effect of their dietary pattern may have been due to several factors: monounsaturated fat (which oxidises less rapidly than polyunsaturates); more natural anti-oxidants (from fruits, vegetables, legumes and wine); or alpha-linolenic acid (usually present in Mediterranean diets as the green leafy vegetable known as purslane). They also noted that since serum cholesterol levels were not significantly different in the experimental or control groups, but no sudden death occurred in the Mediterranean diet group (compared with eight in the control group), the protective effect of their diet may have been the reduction of changes in heart rhythm (arrhythmias), or the lower incidence of platelets clumping together. Such factors are sometimes forgotten when so much emphasis is given to cholesterol. Several studies have shown that omega 3 fatty acids in fish oils reduce arrhythmias in rats and in humans. The Lyon Heart Study's use of the omega 3 alpha-linolenic acid and the Welsh and Norwegian trials support this.

Several other studies using diets with a relatively high content of fat derived largely from nuts (mainly monounsaturated fat) reduced coronary heart disease risk more than diets with less total fat but more polyunsaturated fat.

Those with non-insulin dependent diabetes have a higher than average risk of coronary heart disease. Their diabetes is controlled better if they adopt a diet with more monounsaturated fat compared with one that is low in fat and higher in carbohydrate.

The heart disease diet recommendations have also been complicated by changing opinions about trans fatty acids. Once considered unimportant, the type of trans fatty acids present in the margarines and fats that are used in many processed foods are at least as undesirable as saturated fatty acids. These fats were discussed in greater detail in Chapter 2.

There is now such a body of scientific and medical literature on the subject of diet and heart disease that you can find studies to support many points of view, but not all those studies or points of view are necessarily valid. More than ever it is important to review the subject overall, rather than isolating one aspect.

Some aspects of the links between diet and heart disease have not changed. For example, for adults, it is still desirable to reduce saturated fat. Previous recommendations to increase consumption of polyunsaturated fats, however, are no longer valid. These fats are fine in moderation, but more is not better. Advice on how to reduce the risk of coronary heart disease in adults is to:

- decrease saturated fats;
- select monounsaturated rather than a high intake of polyunsaturated fats;
- ensure an adequate intake of anti-oxidants;
- avoid high levels of trans fatty acids.

Nutrition research tends to divorce nutrients from foods. This can lead to recommendations for dietary patterns that are not found in any cultural cuisine. Had we noted more carefully the diet of healthy populations with low levels of coronary heart disease, we could have found many examples in Asian, Mediterranean and Middle Eastern populations to support each of the points recommended above.

## DIETARY FAT AND CANCER

If we take all cancers together, cancer has now overtaken coronary heart disease as the major cause of death of Australians, according to the Australian Bureau of Statistics. It is also the source of the greatest waste of life, accounting for twice as many years of life lost before age 76 compared with either heart disease or accidents.

Environmental factors are involved in many cancers, although the exact percentages attributable to factors such as cigarette smoking, diet and contact with high levels of various chemical substances are debatable. Most experts agree that about a third of all cancers may be related to what we eat and drink.

The subject of diet and cancer is complex. Many people assume that food additives are the major problems, but more evidence points to fat as the major culprit. Even this is complicated by the fact that a high-fat diet tends to be low in whole grains, fruits and vegetables—foods that contain hundreds of factors that can protect us against many cancer-causing agents. A high-fat diet is also high in total energy and this has been shown in many animal studies to increase the risk of cancer.

It is strange that in countries with bountiful supplies of fruits and vegetables, the consumption of them is dropping. Many people say they don't have time to eat these healthful foods. Instead, encouraged by advertising, they substitute fatty fast foods and takeaway foods, thus giving themselves a double whammy—too much fat and not enough protective food factors. We do not know which is the more relevant to the increasing incidence of some cancers.

In the development of cancers, the transformation of normal cells into malignant ones involves three stages: initiation, promotion and progression. Diet may be involved in all three. Foods may also offer protection against cancer, and what we eat and drink (or fail to eat) may give cells greater (or less) resistance to cancer-causing substances (carcinogens).

The subject of food and cancer is not simple. Carcinogens are sometimes present in foods or may be produced during the cooking or preservation of foods. Fat, or other dietary substances, may also initiate or promote changes in cells or activate carcinogens, while protective factors in foods may deactivate them.

There are many examples of how diet increases the risk of cancer. Epidemiological studies provide the first clues and research then tries to find the specific factors involved, including aspects of diet. They may differ according to the site of each cancer. Some examples of relationships between specific cancers and diet include:

- A high salt intake is related to stomach cancer—now rare in Australia but still the most common cancer throughout the world. It is now thought that a bolus dose of sodium chloride from dried and salted foods, rather than the total daily intake of sodium, is relevant to the damage of cells lining the stomach. A lack of fresh, raw fruits and vegetables is also relevant and deprives the cells of their essential protection.

- A high-fat diet may increase the production of bile acids. Once these have transported partly digested fats into the wall of the intestine, they pass to the large intestine (colon) where they have the potential to cause cancer. A high-fat diet is also usually low in dietary fibre, starch and plant foods and this alters the type and number of colonic bacteria, increases the pH above desirable levels and reduces the production of protective butyrate. With the low faecal bulk and slow transit times caused by a low intake of dietary fibre, any carcinogens will also spend a longer period of time in the colon.

- Alcohol in high doses damages liver cells, increasing their susceptibility to cirrhotic changes and liver cancer.
- Dietary fat, and a high level of body fat, both increase levels of potentially carcinogenic oestrones and oestradiol in post-menopausal women. A high-fibre, low-fat diet, especially one with high quantities of vegetables rich in indoles, alters the chemistry of these compounds so that they are less carcinogenic.

Epidemiological studies indicate strongly that certain types of fat play a role in cancers of the breast, colon, endometrium and prostate. Animal studies back some of these associations. For example, polyunsaturated fatty acids promote carcinogenesis more effectively than saturated fatty acids do, possibly because cancer cells use the essential fatty acid, linoleic acid, as fuel for their own growth.

Such effects have not been noted in human populations, but this is not surprising as they would be difficult to separate from confounding variables. For example, much of the polyunsaturated fat in the Australian diet comes from margarines which also contain compounds such as trans fatty acids and hydrogenated fats, and these compounds are under suspicion.

Fat in the diet may be a major initiator or promoter of cancer. Fat may increase steroid hormones produced in the body or may exert its influence through prostaglandins. It may also affect cell membrane structure and, thus, resistance to carcinogens.

The only fat that has been reported to protect us against cancer is olive oil, although fish oils have been proved successful in experiments with animals. Studies in Greece and Spain have shown a lower incidence of breast cancer in women who consumed olive oil. Many of them used their olive oil to make vegetables more appetising, so it may have been their higher vegetable intake that protected them.

In animals, diets with polyunsaturated fats are more closely associated with cancers in mammary glands and the pancreas, colon, skin and liver than with saturated fats. We cannot apply these studies directly to humans, but they do give some warning signals. It is most likely that specific fatty acids, or the balance of different kinds of fats, may create the greatest risk.

For example, the ratio of omega 6 to omega 3 fatty acids may be relevant. An analysis in 1990 of the large-scale Multiple Risk Factor Intervention Trial conducted in the United States in the 1970s and 1980s showed a strong correlation between the ratio of these two types of polyunsaturated fats and cancer incidence and mortality. In practice, this means that a low intake of fish and vegetables combined with a high intake of polyunsaturated oils and margarines represents a potential hazard for the development of cancer. It is difficult, however, to put the blame wholly on any single food and there is no evidence that polyunsaturated fats themselves cause cancer. They may simply set up the right climate for cancers caused by something else to proliferate. Some studies suggest that too much of any kind of fat may increase the risk of cancer in humans.

One widely publicised United States study maintained that fat was not related to breast cancer, since the incidence of breast cancer in women who had reduced their fat from 40 per cent of kilojoules to 30 per cent did not change. Other researchers have since pointed out that levels of fat may have to go much lower than this before dramatic differences are seen. Epidemiological comparisons of women in Western countries and in Asia suggest that those whose levels of fat fall below 25 per cent of kilojoules (a common percentage throughout Asia) are protected against breast cancer. However, these low levels of fat in the Asian diet are accompanied by a high intake of soy products and vegetables, and it may be these that are giving protection. Asian diets also tend to have low levels of meat.

Epidemiological studies show that those who eat a high-meat diet have higher levels of cancers of the breast, colon, pancreas and prostate. However, it is difficult to separate the effects of meat fat from the meat itself. A high-meat diet may also have fewer vegetables and therefore fewer protective factors. A recent well-conducted Harvard study reported that men who ate red meat as a main dish five or more times a week were 2.6 times as likely to suffer advanced prostate cancer as those who ate red meat once a week or less.

Against these theories, consider also that mammary tumours in rats and stomach and skin cancers in mice are reduced if the animals have a higher level of a fatty acid called conjugated dienoic linoleate (CLA) which occurs in cooked beef and lamb and in heat-treated dairy products such as pasteurised milk, yoghurt and cheeses. CLA seems to have an anti-oxidant role in tissues and is more potent than vitamin E in preventing some reactions related to growth of cancers. It is possible that CLA may compete with and replace less desirable fats trying to get into cell membranes, or it may change messages within cells. Its role is still being explored—we do not yet have all the answers.

The evidence condemning fat, and some foods that contain it, however, continues to grow. High levels of meat protein are under suspicion. Plant foods, by contrast, seem to offer protection against cancer. Milk and yoghurt may also provide some protection against bowel cancer, possibly because of their high content of calcium.

At this stage, the safest advice is to eat more vegetables and other plant foods and less fat, especially fewer omega 6 polyunsaturated fats, unless they are balanced with more of the omega 3 polyunsaturates found in fish and vegetables.

The greatest body of evidence is that fruits and vegetables have cancer protection features. Smokers who eat the most fruit and vegetables are less likely to develop lung cancer compared with smokers who eat fewer fruits and vegetables, and most studies have also shown that cancers of the breast, colon, oesophagus, stomach, pancreas and various other sites have an inverse relationship with fruit and vegetable intake. These foods are major sources of vitamin C and beta carotene, and also have some vitamin E—all anti-oxidant substances. Some researchers jumped to the conclusion that these nutrients protect against cancer, but the results of a recent 8-year Finnish lung cancer trial in which 29,000 smokers were given supplements of these vitamins, either alone or in combination, casts doubt on this simplistic notion. This study showed that no benefit was gained by the supplements and that those taking beta-carotene had a significantly higher incidence of lung cancer. It was a disappointment to those selling vitamin supplements but these findings do not negate the original studies of fruit and vegetables—they may simply contain something else that provides protection.

The National Cancer Institute (NCI) in the United States is working to isolate anti-cancer compounds in fruits and vegetables. It's a long task as there are several thousand compounds to sift through and they estimate that more than 600 may have anti-cancer activity. Other foods including garlic, extra virgin olive oil and chicken also contain anti-cancer compounds. Some compounds have been isolated. For example, broccoli contains sulforaphane, a dithiolthione compound that can block tumour formation in animals. Brussels sprouts, cauliflower, spring onions and cabbage have it too, although in slightly smaller quantities.

It is unlikely that any single substance in fruit and vegetables is providing protection and it is unlikely that the protection will ever be available in a pill. The chances are that many compounds may be involved and that synergistic effects between particular substances are important. At this stage, our only certainty is that eating *more* fruit and vegetables and *less* fat may offer some protection against most of the common cancers, especially bowel cancer. This is almost certainly the diet to which humans are biologically adapted—not the highly processed fatty foods that make up so much of the diet for many people.

## DIETARY FAT AND DIABETES

There is little evidence that the type of diabetes that develops in childhood has anything to do with dietary fat. In this type the body stops producing insulin, the hormone that takes glucose out of the blood and transports it to the cells as a source of energy for them.

The most common form of diabetes, however, is non-insulin dependent diabetes mellitus (or NIDDM), which is increasing rapidly in all developed countries. It is a genetic disease but is strongly related to dietary fat, and most (but not all) cases occur in those who are overweight. If you have the gene for NIDDM but stay slim, exercise regularly and do not consume large quantities of certain fats, the disease will probably never appear.

In NIDDM, the body continues to produce insulin. Sometimes it produces a normal quantity of insulin for a body of normal weight, but it may not be enough for someone who is overweight. Excess quantities of dietary fat can also build up in the membranes around cells so that the insulin cannot get through. This is known as insulin resistance and is characterised by high levels of triglycerides in the bloodstream. In an attempt to overcome the problem, the body produces more insulin, but this still cannot get through. Blood levels of insulin therefore rise. The glucose, meanwhile, is unable to get into the cells so it also builds up in the blood, eventually spilling over into the urine as the body excretes it.

Exercise helps in the treatment of NIDDM as it helps break down the barriers of fat around the cells. Weight loss also helps and the easiest way to accomplish this is to cut back on kilojoules, especially those from sugar, fat and alcohol.

Some recent studies show that diabetes improves if the diet includes a moderate level of fat, mainly monounsaturated fat from a product such as olive oil, plus ample quantities of fish. Most people with diabetes found such a diet easier to stick to than one that had very low levels of fat and more carbohydrate.

After a meal, fats consumed show up in the blood as triglycerides. Some hours later, the triglycerides should have been cleared from the blood and either used for energy or tucked away in fat stores. In NIDDM, high levels of triglycerides are usually still circulating in the blood after an overnight fast.

The treatment for high triglyceride levels is to cut back on saturated fats and reduce the consumption of alcohol and refined sugar. Many researchers also believe it is best to avoid high levels of polyunsaturated fats, and to switch to mono-unsaturates.

## DIETARY FAT AND GALLSTONES

The gall bladder is situated behind the lower ribs on the right side of the body. It stores bile, a golden brown fluid produced by the liver for digesting fats. After a meal, the gall bladder squirts bile into the intestine.

Gallstones form when high levels of cholesterol in bile precipitate and combine with calcium salts to form stones. One or many stones may form, and they can vary from the size of a grain of sand to the size of a golf ball, or even larger.

Gallstones are common in Australia and one in ten men and one in five women develop them. They are more common in older people, in those who are overweight, and in women—especially those who have had many pregnancies. The rate also increases with people who eat a lot of fat, including (some claim *especially*) polyunsaturated fat. A low-fat, high-fibre diet reduces the risk of getting gallstones.

Many people who have gallstones have no symptoms and never develop any. Others have a sudden, severe, steady pain in the upper abdomen which may spread to the chest, shoulders or back and may be accompanied by nausea and vomiting. These symptoms may last for minutes or hours. In some cases, the pain is mild and feels more like indigestion. If a stone blocks the duct that joins the gall bladder to the main bile duct the gall bladder can become inflamed, causing fever and severe pain on the right side of the abdomen. This is called cholecystitis.

No diet or nutritional supplement can dissolve gallstones. During a gallstone attack fatty foods should be avoided, but the pain is related to the attack rather than to specific foods. There is no need to avoid eggs or anything else except high-fat foods.

As gallstones are made in the gall bladder, its removal, along with the stones, will resolve the symptoms and prevent any more stones from developing. Humans can live well without a gall bladder. Bile simply passes from the liver directly to the intestine instead of being stored in the gall bladder. It makes sense, however, not to overdo fatty foods of any kind.

# CHAPTER 4

# Fat and body fat

## HOW MUCH BODY FAT?

Humans need body fat. It pads our joints, and cushions organs such as the kidneys. Body fat also acts as a reserve of fuel to provide energy in times of scarce food supply or illness. Some body fat is also considered aesthetically pleasing, especially in women, possibly because it is a sign of fertility.

## TOO LITTLE BODY FAT

Desirable levels of body fat are influenced by fashion. In modern Western society, most women wish they were thinner. Indoctrinated by media images that a desirable body is lean, many young women go to extreme lengths to minimise their body fat. Many are constantly miserable because they cannot achieve the thinness they consider desirable. Concerns that body fat is ugly have now extended to the absurdity of many normal-weight girls as young as nine or ten developing an intense fear of fat. Athletes and their coaches also want the body pared down to its lean muscle, with as little extra weight to carry as possible. This preoccupation with body weight has increased the incidence of eating disorders. Whereas anorexia nervosa was rarely seen 30 years ago, almost every high school girl now knows at least one victim. Among men eating disorders are still rare, except for male athletes.

Some male athletes strive to reduce fat levels to 4–8 per cent of their body weight. A few runners aim for body fat levels as low as 3 per cent to reduce the load they carry while running, and to get rid of insulation so they can dissipate heat more easily. The equivalent level for female athletes would be 12 per cent body fat. Exercise physiologists warn that such low levels of body fat, in men or women, pose the danger of a reduced capacity for exercise and greater likelihood of injury and illness.

Most women stop menstruating when body fat levels fall. At least 16 per cent fat is needed for menstruation to occur at all, and approximately 22 per cent body fat is usually needed for a regular menstrual cycle. At lower levels of body fat ovulation may occur only occasionally, so those female athletes who do not menstruate but don't want to become pregnant must take contraceptive precautions.

While lack of fertility may not concern an actively competing athlete, the low levels of oestrogen that accompany it result in a loss of calcium from bone. Such losses usually occur at menopause, when oestrogen supplies normally fall and the risk of osteoporosis increases dramatically. Ten years after menstruation ceases, 60 per cent of women have substantial loss of bone density. In Australia and most Western countries, one woman in four will have a serious bone fracture of the hip or spine after menopause. The longer women live, the greater their bone loss and the higher their chance of a serious fracture. The best prevention is to build a strong skeleton early in life when more calcium can be absorbed into bone, and then maintain this with a good level of calcium and physical activity.

The process of bone loss begins at whatever age women are when they stop menstruating. Studies on bone density of female athletes show alarming levels of osteoporosis, even while they are in their late teen years and early twenties. No amount of exercise or calcium intake can protect them against such high calcium losses while their hormone levels are low.

Young women need to build dense bones to withstand the inevitable losses associated with ageing after menopause. Very thin young women, whether athletes or not, have a double problem. Not only do they begin to lose bone density many years earlier than other women do, but they miss the opportune time during their younger years to build up bone density. The best prevention against osteoporosis is to keep body fat levels at least normal, or slightly above normal to maintain hormone levels, and to maintain an adequate calcium intake and some weight-bearing exercise.

It is ironic that many young women diet to reduce body fat to look more attractive, yet the loss of bone density that accompanies their slenderness will cause a stooped, painful posture within 10 to 20 years. A young woman of 17 who reduces her body fat level enough for her periods to cease may think she looks attractive now, but she can expect to spend much of her life looking *less* attractive than those carrying more fat but possessing a straight, strong spine.

Although percentage body fat has begun to dominate the thinking of many men and women in countries such as Australia, it is very hard to measure it accurately. Many fitness centres and gymnasiums use callipers to estimate skinfold thickness at various body sites and then use a formula to calculate body fat. Skinfold measurements are notoriously difficult to take accurately, and the formula has been discredited for its inaccuracy. This has not stopped people quoting body fat levels determined by these methods. Underwater weighing or computed tomography (CT scanning) can measure body fat more accurately, but these are expensive techniques not readily available to most people. It seems more sensible to stop quoting body fat percentages. If fitness centres and gymnasiums would help by no longer using such flawed measurements and formulas, many people may be less likely to dwell on exact body fat percentage and think more about keeping the body in basic good shape.

## TOO MUCH BODY FAT

It is undesirable to be too thin, but it is also hazardous to be too fat, especially if the excess fat is around the waist and on the upper body. A certain level of body fat is essential for the adequate production of female hormones, but there does not seem to be a similar role for extra fat on men. Excess fat on males is deposited in fat stores in the abdomen, known as visceral fat. There is a strong body of evidence that this fat is a health hazard, increasing the risk of coronary heart disease, high blood pressure, diabetes and bowel cancer.

Overweight men were rare in most societies until recent times, when the food supply had become assured and physical effort was no longer necessary to collect food. Since machinery has been used for most physically demanding tasks, and most men drive cars instead of walking or cycling, the number with excess visceral fat has increased dramatically. In Australia there are far more over-fat men than women, although the opposite is true in the United States. By their mid-thirties, 40 per cent of Australian men are fatter than is healthy and this rises to more than 50 per cent by age 50.

Up to age 40, few women in Australia are too fat and being underweight is more common than being overweight. During their forties and fifties, however, women, too, succumb to excess body fat. Many women think this has something to do with changing hormone levels, but it is more likely because they are less physically active once their children have grown up. Caring for children and the extra household tasks they create uses up energy, so that when these physical demands are no longer required women tend to gain body fat. When children leave home, many women also eat out more. Few older women exercise regularly, so their total energy expenditure goes down while their input increases.

Body fat begins to accumulate slowly some years before menopause but it is not until 4 or 5 kilos have settled that most women realise that this weight gain has become a permanent part of their body. This realisation usually coincides with menopause, which is then blamed. Women gain much the same amount of weight whether or not they use hormone replacement therapy—more evidence that the weight gain has more to do with ageing and reduced physical activity than with changing hormone levels.

In affluent countries, high levels of body fat

in both sexes and all ages are due to a lack of exercise and a modern food supply that is high in fat. Only eating fat causes fat to be deposited in the first place, although once excess fat is in place, kilojoules from any source will prevent its loss. The average Westerner admits to eating about 100 grams of fat a day and almost certainly consumes more. Studies show that most people underestimate their food intake, and overweight people underestimate more than those of normal weight do. Since fat hit the headlines as being undesirable, most people are even less likely to report their true intake, so that finding out how much fat people really eat is now difficult.

In surveys where people are given a list of foods and asked to mark how often they eat each of them (known as Food Frequency Questionnaires), even those trying to fill out such forms accurately find it difficult. Many foods are not mentioned and few people eat the same meals and snacks every day. The best of the Food Frequency lists contain about 180 different foods. The average Australian supermarket stocks around 15,000 items, and in Europe and the United States there are even more. A product not listed may contribute only 0.5 per cent of the dietary fat, but if there are many such foods the estimation is highly inaccurate. The fact that one third of the food dollar is now spent on foods prepared outside the home also distorts figures. Almost invariably, people assume that such foods have a composition similar to those they would prepare themselves, whereas nearly all foods cooked on commercial premises have fat levels higher than those prepared in the home kitchen.

The difficulty of measuring what people really eat has resulted in survey reports claiming that average fat consumption is going down, even though the population is growing steadily fatter. This does not make sense, even allowing for changes in physical activity. Comparing physical activity in the 1950s with the 1980s shows a big fall, but little significant difference since then. Yet from the 1980s to the mid-1990s, the average person in the Australian population gained about a gram of fat a day.

Food frequency data represent a wish list of what people think they *should* be eating, not the true consumption facts. Sales figures for fast foods, takeaways, crisps, chips, chocolates, croissants, cakes and pastries all show increases. Meanwhile, sales figures for fruit and vegetables are falling as people omit them in favour of the fatty food range. The facts are that fat consumption is increasing and is raising our body fat levels.

## WHAT MAKES YOU FAT?

Nutritionists once believed that too many kilojoules

from any source would add to body fat. We now know that this is not true. Proteins are not stored and are rarely converted to fat and the body is not able to convert alcohol to fat.

Until recently, carbohydrates have born the brunt of the blame for excess body fat but research from several laboratories now confirms their innocence. The body does not store much carbohydrate, apart from some stored in muscles as glycogen and a smaller quantity as liver glycogen. Some carbohydrate goes to replenish blood glucose levels and the rest stimulates the body to burn more energy. Humans don't convert carbohydrate to fat until the intake exceeds 500 grams—the amount in 32 slices of bread, 11 cups of cooked rice, or almost 4 kilograms of potatoes! The old idea that eating an extra 100 g potato every day for 40 days would add a kilogram of fat is not true. You would have to eat 40 extra potatoes in one day! However, a daily excess of 800 kilojoules (190 calories) from fat can produce such a gain over a month.

In practice, humans do not get fat from eating carbohydrate-rich foods, *unless* those foods have added fat, which can be converted to body fat. This is different from the situation in other animals where carbohydrates are readily converted to fat. But then, few animals eat a diet high in fat. Even carnivorous animals, who eat only animal flesh, will not get much fat if the animals they are eating are wild.

By contrast, many of the foods we eat—including many carbohydrate-rich foods—are high in fat. Bread, rice, potatoes and pasta have little fat, but we put butter or margarine on the bread, fry the rice, add sour cream or butter to potatoes, or fry them in fat to make chips or crisps, and smother pasta in either creamy sauces or add loads of fatty meat and cheese. Many people then blame the bread, rice, potatoes or pasta for making them fat. It is not necessary to restrict carbohydrate foods unless they are also high in fat.

With the exception of sugar, foods high in carbohydrate are also bulky and this effectively restricts consumption. Carbohydrate-rich foods also regulate the appetite whereas foods rich in fat do not.

Because alcohol is toxic to the body, it will always be used as fast as the body can oxidise it and extract its kilojoules. We burn the kilojoules from alcohol first and then use up carbohydrates and proteins. Only then does the body get round to burning up fats.

This does *not* mean that the kilojoules from beer or wine or bread don't count. These foods don't add to body fat but their kilojoules are relevant for those who don't want to gain more fat, or for those who want to lose the fat they already have. Consuming large quantities of alcohol or any carbohydrate food can supply enough kilojoules for all the body's energy needs so that it has no need to burn fat from either the last meal or the stores waiting around the waist.

Almost all chronic alcoholics who have a high kilojoule intake from alcohol, but eat little food, are thin. In spite of this, most people cling to the idea that the typical beer gut is due to beer. Some people of both sexes believe that a beer gut is some kind of a swollen stomach. They fail to realise that paunches of all sizes are composed of fat. They also do not think to lay the blame where it belongs—on the food that is usually consumed with beer.

Most beer drinkers eat fatty foods with their beer—peanuts, cabanossi sausage, salamis, cheese and biscuits, sausage rolls, meat pies, hamburgers, fatty barbecues and large untrimmed steaks. It is rare to find anyone using the amber liquid to wash down a green salad!

The reason why many hearty drinkers get fat is that the fuel provided by alcohol is enough for their needs. Any kilojoules from fat consumed at the same time are therefore surplus and are deposited as body fat—usually around the waist. A beer gut should more correctly be called a *fat gut*.

## FAT MAKES FAT

Research now shows conclusively that fat in the

diet is the major culprit in producing body fat. The body can store large amounts of fat. It is the last priority as a fuel for metabolism or physical activity. Eating more fat does not increase the amount of fat oxidised and fat has little effect in satiating appetite. A diet high in fat leads to passive and chronic over-consumption, and increases the store of body fat.

There are now many studies showing that body fat correlates with fat intake, not specifically with kilojoule intake. Of course, since fats have more than twice the kilojoule level of either carbohydrates or proteins, and a higher level than alcohol, a diet high in fat is usually high in kilojoules. It is not the kilojoules themselves that are to blame, but their source.

Australians eat a lot of fat. In spite of moves to low-fat dairy products and encouragement to trim fat from meat, fat consumption is still high, largely because of the high quantities of fat used in fast foods, processed foods and ready-made meals.

Few people realise that they are eating a lot of fat. Many *think* they are eating less fat by consuming meals they consider 'light'. The composition of such foods shows they are not light in fat. For example, a slice of quiche with salad can have six times the fat levels of lean meat and vegetables; and a typical helping of lasagne or a coconut-based Thai curry have far more fat than a traditional roast dinner. Few people realise that a modern hamburger contains 30 grams of fat compared with the 18 grams of the old-fashioned variety, or that spaghetti bought from a takeaway store has had every one of its strands of spaghetti coated in fat to prevent them sticking together and contains a rich cream-based sauce to boot! Ready-prepared meals almost always have more fat than home-cooked meals.

The influx of reduced-fat foods doesn't always help. There is some evidence that people maintain a liking for fat when they eat fat-reduced foods but lose their taste for it if they eat very little of it. Many reduced-fat products are still relatively high in fat. For example, reduced-fat margarines may have 60 per cent fat, reduced-fat cheeses range from 7 to 25 per cent fat (regular cheddar is 33 per cent fat), and some reduced-fat pies and meals are still high in fat. Each of these products may have less fat than its regular counterpart, but is still high in fat. Being labelled as 'reduced-fat', however, may make people feel free to consume larger quantities. For example, those who might hesitate to eat even one scoop of regular ice-cream each night may feel quite comfortable about frequently having two scoops of reduced-fat ice cream. It is a bit like seeing someone putting skim milk in their coffee while scoffing apple pie with cream.

We need to know where fats are. We also need

to understand that we do not need to remove *all* fat from the diet—less will do nicely—and that we can still allow foods to maintain flavour. In fact, it also makes good sense to use foods with plenty of flavour. For example, a teaspoon of a well-flavoured olive oil will add more flavour to a salad than a tablespoon of a bland oil can, and a small sprinkle of good Parmesan cheese will give as much flavour as a much larger quantity of mild cheese.

Some carbohydrate-rich foods are valuable because they are filling—especially potatoes. Most carbohydrate foods are served with something fatty, but there are alternatives. Here are some examples:

- Crisp up good-quality bread or rolls in a hot oven, or buy when very fresh so they taste good without a spread.
- Try pita and lavash breads with salad or hommos and tabouli, or with a variety of other ingredients.
- Dollop low-fat yoghurt mixed with fresh snipped herbs on top of potatoes in place of butter.
- Serve or order steamed rice rather than fried rice.
- Make sauces for pasta by mixing a small amount of olive oil with low-fat ingredients such as tomatoes, mushrooms, eggplant,

onions, garlic, capsicum, herbs, wine, seafood, chicken breast or very lean meat.

- Serve well-chilled, fresh fruit in season, without cream or ice-cream but with yoghurt, if desired.

## FAT LOSS

Excess fat accumulates because the kilojoules entering the body from food and drink exceed the amount required for growth, physical activity and metabolism. The only way to lose body fat is to create a kilojoule deficit until the excess fat is lost and then establish a balance between what comes in and what is used.

Most people who are too fat are convinced they have some kind of deficiency in their metabolism. Many studies show this is rarely the case. The problem of excess body fat is almost always due to over-consumption and under-activity. Those who diet frequently, however, may reduce the kilojoules they need for metabolism because most diets reduce lean tissue rather than fat, and lean tissue is what burns up kilojoules 24 hours a day.

Genetics are involved in excess weight, and this field is still being explored. Experts say, however, that genes are responsible for only one-quarter to one-third of excess weight. Environmental factors such as food, drink and exercise are still the major weight contributors.

There is a common misconception that some people are fortunate enough never to gain weight. In fact, everyone will gain weight if overfed, but some will gain more than others. Many of those who seem to eat a lot but stay slim tend to eat more when others are present but do not have a high intake all the time. Some are natural fidgets who burn up more than 3000 kilojoules a day just in their constant body movements.

For those who need to lose body fat there are some suggestions that might be useful, but note first these three important points:

- Not everyone is going to be the same size. No amount of dieting will give you sylph-like thighs if they don't run in your family. Remember that the health hazard is fat around the waist and on the upper body.
- Fast weight loss is not fat loss but represents mainly changes in the body's content of water, and some loss of lean tissue. Weight lost fast usually returns, often bringing a bonus kilo or two.
- Changes in eating and exercise must be upheld forever, not just for three weeks nor even three months or three years. Such changes therefore must be possible, sustainable and enjoyable.

The best way to create a kilojoule deficit is by eating less fat and doing more exercise to burn it up. Try also to reduce sugar and alcohol. Neither will add to body fat, but neither provide essential elements and both provide energy which the body could otherwise get from its fat stores. Trying to cut out sugar and alcohol, however, is not a good tactic, as forbidden foods become highly desirable. An occasional cake, chocolate, ice-cream, or whatever sweet food you like makes good sense. Make sure it is worth the kilojoules by choosing an exceptional cake or chocolate rather than something mundane. You must also make sure that your 'occasions' don't come more than once or twice a week.

A daily glass of wine or a single beer won't usually interfere with successful fat loss, but don't consume it fast to satisfy thirst. No alcoholic beverage is a good thirst quencher, so always drink plenty of water *before* starting on any type of alcohol. Drinking one or two large glasses of water first is the most painless way to reduce alcohol consumption.

There is little point in cutting down on bulky carbohydrate foods. They have the great advantage of being filling. Most people can put up with feeling hungry for a day or so, but after that they become very hungry and less discriminating about what they eat. Many studies show that strict dieting leads to eating binges and greater consumption of high-fat foods. It makes more sense to eat foods such as potatoes, breads, cereals and other grain products, as well as plenty of fruit and vegetables. Eating fruit with fibre instead of drinking juice and eating high-fibre bread also helps to make you feel more satisfied.

Very strict diets don't work. Apart from the difficulty in sticking to them, eating very little carbohydrate leads to a loss of water and lean tissue and reduces the body's energy expenditure. Water losses can be replaced, but lean tissue burns up kilojoules and its loss eventually leads to weight gain. The body's spontaneous reduction in energy expenditure, when running on a very low-kilojoule diet, is also counterproductive. Eating very little and having low energy levels just makes you feel awful.

## FATS IN FOOD

In the Australian diet, the major contributors to fat intake are fats and oils, meat and dairy products. Fats and oils are used in the home for cooking and as spreads for bread. An even greater quantity come in processed and takeaway foods. Many fast foods are obviously fatty, leaving grease on your fingers. Others hide their fat in soft buns, meat patties coated with cheese and fatty dressings added to make the product more moist so that it can be eaten more quickly. Among Asian takeaway foods, fried noodles, fried rice, battered foods and sauces that include coconut milk also contribute a lot of fat. Other high-fat foods include margarine, chips, crisps and savoury snack foods, biscuits (including savoury crackers), chocolate and some other types of confectionery, cheeses, cream, cakes, pastries, pies, croissants and creamy sauces.

The high-fat content of food eaten outside the home comes not only from the ingredients, but also from the larger-than-average serving sizes. This is more apparent at the lower price end of the market. Somewhat ironically, as you pay more you get less. In the United States, serving sizes are something of a joke to the rest of the world. A food or drink marked 'small' is akin to something regarded as 'giant-sized' in other countries. This undoubtedly contributes to the high level of obesity in the United States.

Whether snacking is involved in weight gain is debatable. When given a set amount of food as either meals or snacks, most people burn more kilojoules with the snacks. In practice, however, most people eat snacks in addition to their normal meals and these become extra sources of fat and kilojoules.

Perhaps the best example of the wisdom of avoiding snacks comes from France. Obesity is uncommon in France, even though the French people seem to eat many foods that the rest of the world regards as undesirable—for example, cheese and butter. Overall, the French do not snack a lot. Meals are taken so seriously that casual eating while walking along the street or driving in a car is less common than in countries such as the United States where meals and snacks mingle freely throughout the day. It is possible that the habit of eating discreet meals allows the body to digest one lot of food and feel hungry before eating another. That is, this habit may allow the body's natural appetite control mechanism to work better than it does when we eat food merely in response to the sight of it.

To lose body fat, most people will achieve the best success if they restrict their daily fat intake to 30 to 40 grams a day. Some steps to achieve this might include:

## Skip spreads

For the average person, skipping margarine and butter will save about 20 grams of fat a day. For big consumers, who are likely to be overweight, the saving will be even greater. In a recent study where people were asked to keep their total fat to 30 to 40 grams a day and were given a list of the fat content of foods but no other instructions, every person spontaneously decided that one of the easiest ways to reduce fat intake was to stop using margarine or butter. But changing to a reduced-fat spread does not usually work because most people simply use more. It takes only a week or so to become used to avoiding spreads. Eating bread with no spread is widely practised in most Mediterranean countries where bread consumption is two to four times greater than that of countries such as Australia. It must therefore be possible, and almost certainly enjoyable.

## Eat fewer takeaway foods

Most people used to eat fast foods and takeaway meals only occasionally. They now account for one third of the money spent on food—even more in some countries. Almost without exception, fast foods are fatty and carry much higher fat levels than home-cooked foods do. For example, a modern burger has 30 grams of fat; add another 20 grams if you eat it with a medium serve of French fries. Fried chicken is no better and even a small slice of ready-made quiche carries 25 grams of fat. Add a salad with dressing and you've easily exceeded the day's 30 gram fat total in one small meal.

Adults and teenagers are now being wooed to eat fast food breakfasts too. This is another disaster, with a full breakfast adding 34 grams of fat and even scrambled egg and muffin contributing 21 grams. Compare this with the total of 3 grams you get in a bowl of cereal with non-fat milk, some fresh fruit and a slice of toast with marmalade.

Fast food meals are seen as being quick, convenient and relatively cheap, yet many meals can be prepared in 15 or 20 minutes at home from ingredients that can be stored in the pantry, fridge and freezer and cost less than the total amount spent at a fast-food restaurant. Some examples of quick and easy meals are listed further on in the chapter.

# Eat bread instead of biscuits, pastries or croissants

Two average slices of bread or a fresh bread roll each have 1.5 grams of fat. A croissant has as much fat as 19 slices of bread! A small pastry is similar. Biscuits add up too. Six small crackers have 6 grams of fat, two small cream-filled biscuits have 7 grams of fat. Chocolate-coated biscuits have even more. Nibbling a few biscuits with every cup of tea or coffee can add up to a hefty fat total.

## Cut fat off meat and chicken

Two lamb chops with fat have 30 grams of fat; trimmed of most external fat they have 11 grams. Very lean meats now available have a low fat content and most cuts of chicken can now be found already skinned.

## Choose low-fat milk and yoghurt

This is one of the easiest changes for most people.

There is little to be gained from changing to low-fat milk for the slurp added to tea or coffee, especially if you don't like its taste in these beverages, but it does reduce fat intake if you use it on cereal, in cappuccinos and in cooking.

## Use plenty of ingredients to add flavour to foods

Herbs, spices, lemon, garlic, pepper and wine have no fat, but adding them to food cooked without a lot of fat makes it taste much better. Extra virgin olive oil can also add lots of flavour to a meal, but each teaspoon has 5 grams of fat, so always use it sparingly. All varieties of olive oil, including light oil, have the same fat and kilojoule level as any other oil.

In practice, you can keep fat to 30 to 40 grams, assuming servings are average size, as follows:

| Food | Fat content (g) |
| --- | --- |
| Fruit, 3–6 pieces | <1 |
| Vegetables, 4–5 types | <1 |
| Bread, 6 slices | 4 |
| Breakfast cereal, 1 bowl | 2 |
| Skim milk or non-fat yoghurt | 0* |
| Regular milk in tea or coffee | 4 |
| Rice or pasta, average serve | 2 |
| Egg, cheese, chicken or avocado on sandwich | 6 |
| Lean meat or chicken, average serve | 8** |

| Food | Fat content (g) |
|---|---|
| Olive oil (in cooking), 1 teaspoon | 5 |
| *Total* | *33* |

\*    *If using 200 mL reduced-fat milk, add 3*

\*\*   *Substituting grilled or barbecued seafood reduces this to 2–6 grams*

# EASY LOW-FAT MEAL SUGGESTIONS, ALL BASED ON AVERAGE-SIZED SERVINGS

*Breakfasts* (all with 3–4 grams of fat)

- Cereal with fresh fruit, low-fat milk or yoghurt plus 1 slice of toast with honey, jam or marmalade.
- Smoothie made with low-fat milk, 1–2 bananas, honey and wheatgerm.
- Baked beans on 1 slice of toast.
- Sweet corn, grilled tomatoes and grilled mushrooms on 2 slices of toast.

*Lunch* (all less than 7 grams of fat)

- Sandwiches with salad, sliced turkey and cranberry sauce, plus 1–2 pieces of fruit.
- Pita bread with salad and lean chicken, plus 1 piece of fruit.
- Smoked salmon or tuna mixed with chopped celery and low-fat yoghurt plus 1 bread roll, plus fruit.

- Home-made pumpkin, bean or vegetable soup with 1 bread roll, plus fruit.
- Baked beans on 2 slices of toast.
- Large salad with hard-boiled egg or lean beef, bread roll, plus one or two pieces of fruit.

*Dinner* (all less than 10–15 grams of fat, if cooked with very little oil)

- Spaghetti with sauce made from tomatoes, garlic, mushrooms, capsicum, eggplant, herbs and red wine, plus a green salad dressed with balsamic vinegar and a few drops of olive oil.
- Stir-fried pork with vegetables and rice.
- Lean grilled beef or kangaroo steak with potato and vegetables.
- Grilled fish, steamed or microwaved potatoes with parsley and chives and steamed or microwaved vegetables or salad.
- Couscous with grilled herbed chicken breast and vegetables stir-fried in a little olive oil.
- Lasagne made with spinach, tuna and low-fat ricotta, plus a green salad.

*Dessert*: fresh fruit of any kind, with low-fat yoghurt if desired

*Snacks* (all less than 2 grams of fat)

- Fresh fruit of any kind.
- Fresh bread (just buy a roll and eat it straight).
- Milkshake made with low-fat milk, ice, low-

fat yoghurt, a little honey and coffee, vanilla or fresh fruit for flavour.

- A carton of low-fat yoghurt.
- Breakfast cereal with low-fat milk.
- A couple of rice crackers with honey or banana.

## FRYING IN FAT

All fried foods absorb some fat. As discussed in chapter 2, some oils should not be used more than once for frying because heat causes undesirable chemical changes in them. There are some misconceptions about frying, however, the greatest being that shallow-fried food absorbs less fat than deep-fried food.

The amount of fat absorbed depends on the type of food, the oil and the frying temperature. The National Heart Foundation in Australia has found that potato chips deep-fried at 180–185°C absorb 30 per cent less fat than those cooked at lower temperatures. Thick chips absorb less fat than thin French fries do. And Spanish and Italian researchers report that if you deep-fry in olive oil, less oil is absorbed into foods.

Most commercial deep-fried food is cooked in a highly saturated mixture of palm, palm kernel and hydrogenated soy or cottonseed oils. It may taste good, but it is a disaster for health and weight.

Polyunsaturated oils are not suitable for deep-frying as they are easily degraded by heat and can form undesirable compounds. Using a little polyunsaturated oil to stop food sticking to a pan won't cause problems, but if it is used for deep-frying the leftover oil should be thrown out. This can cause environmental problems if released into the sewerage system, so it should probably be tipped into soil. The simplest solution is probably not to use it at all for deep-frying.

# CHAPTER 5

# Fat-free fats

## THE MARKET FOR FAKE FATS

Almost everyone now knows that fats are fattening. Some are also aware that certain fats can contribute to heart disease, high blood pressure, diabetes, gallstones and some cancers. Yet most people throughout the world are consuming more and more foods high in fat. For some, high-fat foods are such an intrinsic part of their diet that they cannot consider going without them. Many of these people are now looking for foods that look and taste as though they are rich in fat, but have little or none of the genuine article.

The food industry has therefore spent millions of dollars and years of research trying to come up with fat-free fat. They want something that looks like fat, rolls around in the mouth like fat, slips down the throat creamily as fat does—but does not have the kilojoules that normal fats provide.

The market for fat replacers and fake fats is growing rapidly. Most begin in the United States where, between 1986 and 1990, new products which claimed to be *low* or *no fat* grew from a tiny

0.5 per cent of new products to over 11 per cent. Since 1990, the market has grown even more rapidly. By the year 2000, annual sales of reduced-fat margarines, salad and cooking oils alone are expected to exceed $US500 million. If we included no-fat yoghurts, creams, ice-creams, cookies, crisps, chips and other snack foods, chocolate, crackers, biscuits, cakes, pies, pastries, frozen confections, packet sauces, dressings, entrees, main dinners and desserts—all made with fake fats— the figure would balloon. Despite the plethora of such products, however, people of all ages and both sexes in the United States continue to grow fatter.

Australia is following suit, with increasing levels of obesity and more foods containing fat substitutes. At this stage, Australians are much less overweight than Americans, and can buy only a fraction of the no-fat products available in the United States. Some might never be accepted. For example, it is unlikely that Australians would buy the no-fat sour cream labelled 'all natural' that is available in the United States. Not one of its long list of ingredients had any relationship to a cow, and many Australians not used to seeing 15 or 20 ingredients listed on a label would probably be turned off the product.

With an increasing percentage of the population becoming overweight, however, and more people feeling paranoid about all fat, there is a strong chance that more such products could become common throughout the developed world.

## OLESTRA

Not long ago, a top chef in the United States prepared a meal of thick seafood soup, herb-crusted fried duck breast, fried trout, fried soft-shell crayfish, salad with vinaigrette dressing and a rich cake. Each dish was prepared with lots of oil. Such a meal would usually contain more than 100 grams of fat. In this meal, however, each dish was prepared with olestra, an oil made from a fake fat that is one of a range of such foods permitted in the United States. The fat content of this experimental olestra-rich meal was minimal.

At the time of writing, olestra had not been approved for use as a cooking fat in any country in the world. In the United States, it is limited to a range of snack foods, the most popular being potato crisps and similar savoury snacks. Olestra is not yet used at all in Europe and Australia, and many nutritionists and consumer advocates hope it won't be given a green light because it could be one of the biggest disasters ever to hit our food supply.

Technically, olestra is known as a sucrose polyester, sometimes written as SPE, and just like any polyester it is a molecule manufactured in a laboratory. It does not occur naturally. Fats are usually made up of triglycerides—three fatty acid molecules attached to a form of alcohol known as glycerol, as described in chapter 2. Olestra was developed when scientists began tinkering with the number of fatty acids and discovered that an increase in fatty acids decreased the body's ability to digest and absorb the fat. By linking six or eight fatty acids to an alcohol group, joined in turn to a ring of sucrose (sugar) molecules, they came up with a sucrose polyester which they called olestra. The molecules are large and so compact that normal fat-splitting enzymes in the intestine can't get at them.

Unlike some other substitute products, olestra has a wide range of uses including frying, spreading on toast, or as a fat replacement ingredient in crisps, chips, pizzas, fast foods, snack foods, biscuits, pastries, cakes, desserts, confectionery, ice-creams, sauces, mayonnaise and margarine. It has no flavour of its own but in foods it attracts flavours in much the same way other fats do. In the mouth, it tastes like an oil.

The texture, taste and mouthfeel are remarkably like many other processed tasteless fats, although those with a sensitive palate can detect foods that are cooked in olestra. The newspaper *USA Today* asked 44 people who happened to be passing by to taste potato crisps cooked either in olestra or in the usual fat. They were not told which was which, but 25 people correctly identified the crisps cooked in olestra. Many thought the difference was slight and few objected. While this did not involve enough people to make it scientifically valid, it is always interesting to see spontaneous tests done by ordinary people and not by someone trying to market a product.

Because olestra is not recognised by human digestive enzymes, it passes through the body without contributing any kilojoules or cholesterol. That sounds ideal but olestra's passage through the gastrointestinal tract can cause problems. Some of these, such as bloating, abdominal pain and loose stools, may appear within hours of eating it, while for others it may take 20 to 30 years to become apparent. It is these long-term effects that worry many nutritionists.

In some people, olestra passes to the large bowel to be excreted along with other waste products. In others, it may simply ooze through the digestive system and be discharged when you least expect it. The company making olestra has spent a lot of time and money, and has changed the viscosity of the product to reduce the likelihood of this problem. The product in its oil form now looks rather like vaseline. In spite of the changes, however, the US Food and Drug Administration (FDA) still requires products containing olestra to carry a warning that 'olestra may cause abdominal cramping and loose stools'.

Olestra's manufacturers claim that only a small percentage of people suffer undesirable gastrointestinal effects, but this is disputed by some researchers who believe that this percentage is larger. The quantity consumed will obviously have some influence on the potential problem, and if such fake fats are added to a wide variety of foods, or used in excessive quantities as described in the meal at the beginning of this chapter, a much higher percentage of people are likely to suffer abdominal cramping and loose stools.

In test studies where people were given 32 grams of olestra a day in muffins, dinner rolls and other foods, almost one-quarter developed diarrhoea. Other informal surveys gave people a small serving of potato crisps that contained either regular fat or olestra, without the recipients knowing which type they were getting. None of those who had regular crisps had gastrointestinal changes whereas one-sixth of those whose potato crisps contained olestra had bloating or loose stools.

I am less concerned about abdominal effects because at least they will stop most people who experience them from consuming any more products containing olestra. More serious is the fact that on its way through the gastrointestinal tract, olestra may also take with it the fat soluble vitamins A, D, E and K. In the United States, the manufacturers of olestra, to their credit, have been concerned about this and are adding these vitamins to snack foods that contain olestra. The FDA requires a label statement on foods telling consumers that 'olestra inhibits the absorption of some vitamins and other nutrients. Vitamins A, D, E and K have been added'.

The major problem is that vitamins A and D are potentially dangerous in excess. If olestra is added to a broader range of foods, how can we control the total dose? Too much vitamin A is especially hazardous in pregnancy and has been shown to increase the risk of deformities in the foetus. That's why vitamin manufacturers have either removed vitamin A from multivitamins or reduced the amount, and must legally include a warning about possible danger for pregnant women. Vitamin D is also dangerous in excess. It therefore does not make sense to add these vitamins to a wide range of foods.

It is difficult to take in too much of these vitamins from natural sources because they are found in a rather limited number of foods, and usually not in large quantities. The richest source of vitamin A is liver, and some medical authorities think pregnant women should avoid it just in case some eat an excessive quantity. The chances of over-consuming foods such as potato crisps, snack foods and desserts containing olestra and added vitamin A would be much greater. All products with olestra and added vitamin A should therefore carry a warning that they must not be consumed by pregnant women. Young children might also need some restriction of their vitamin A intake.

Vitamin D normally comes from the action of sunlight on a substance in skin. Tanning of the skin exerts a natural control over excess vitamin D being made in this way because it slows the reaction. Adding vitamin D to foods, however, is potentially hazardous. Just five to ten times the Recommended Daily Intake (RDI) is dangerous. Olestra can cause substantial losses of vitamin D from the body, but if the fake fat was used in many foods, and each had extra vitamin D to make up for the losses olestra causes, it would be virtually impossible to control the intake of vitamin D. Even if the product's label recommended limits on how much of it consumers of different ages and sizes should eat, the total vitamin D intake would depend on how many foods containing olestra were consumed each day. In practice, adding vitamin D to a range of foods is not feasible. For this reason alone, some people consider olestra is a hazard in the food supply.

Potentially, there is an even more serious problem. Olestra can also remove from the body some of the protective carotenoid substances occurring in fruit and vegetables. There is strong evidence that these substances function as anti-cancer agents, protecting DNA from the damage that increases the risks of many types of cancer.

More than 200 studies have shown that those who eat the most fruit and vegetables have the lowest incidence of cancer at almost every site in the body. Over 50 studies have specifically shown that diets rich in the wide variety of carotenoids found in fruits and vegetables are associated with a lower risk of cancers.

The best known carotenoid is beta carotene, often called pro-vitamin A, which the body converts to vitamin A. Until recently, other carotenoids were largely ignored because they do not form vitamin A and were therefore thought to have no benefit for humans. Researchers have recently found that these other carotenoids in fruit and vegetables protect against some cancers, whereas beta-carotene may not do so.

Two major trials, in which beta-carotene was given as a supplement, found an *increase* in the incidence of lung cancer, and two other trials have found an increase in bowel polyps, the precursors to bowel cancer. There is some evidence that a carotenoid called lycopene may give protection against cancer but even this is an educated guess, not proof. We really do not know which of the carotenoids in fruit and vegetables give the best protection. We may need all, or at least many of them, and singling out just one is no guarantee of safety. Health authorities therefore unanimously recommend that we increase our consumption of a variety of fruit and vegetables.

The anti-cancer compounds in fruit and vegetables don't make us immune to cancer but they help the body's immune system fight cancer-causing substances that come from cigarette smoking, pollution and, possibly, too much of some kinds of fat. They also protect against coronary heart disease and cataracts, and other eye problems associated with ageing.

Many of the carotenoids need some fat for their absorption. For example, lycopene, which occurs in tomatoes and watermelons and protects against prostate cancer, is absorbed better from a meal that also contains some fat. Using a fake fat, such as olestra, may interfere directly with the absorption of lycopene, and also reduce absorption because it has been substituted for a real fat.

You may not need much olestra to wipe out the value of carotenoids. Researchers in the Netherlands recently reported that small quantities of olestra significantly depleted these natural protective agents. They included modest quantities of olestra in a margarine and measured the effect on five different carotenoids and vitamin E levels in the body. Their report stated that 'even at low doses, sucrose polyester strongly reduces plasma carotenoid concentrations'. Olestra's supporters don't consider there is enough proof that carotenoids are valuable natural anti-cancer substances. It would take decades of research to prove they are wrong and we cannot gamble with people's lives and health in this way.

Two carotenoids, lutein and xeathanthin, are also important in the macula of the eye, the region that permits us to see fine detail. Degeneration of the macula is the major cause of partial visual impairment and blindness that accompanies old age. Studies have already shown that those with low levels of these two carotenoids in their blood have a much greater risk of developing macula degeneration and blindness.

We simply don't know what the long-term effects of olestra are. We do know that, so far, it has reduced the body's levels of every carotenoid tested. As there are more than 600 of these substances, complete test results are almost impossible. We must question whether a food company should have the right to add something to foods that may turn out to have such profoundly dreadful effects on health, especially when the substance is being added only so that people can stuff themselves with more food than their bodies need.

Unlike other food additives, olestra is not taken into the body in milligram or microgram doses but in grams—hundreds or even thousands of times the dose of most food additives. Every substance known is toxic if the dose is large enough.

If olestra is allowed to be used in a wide range of products, most would be marketed as guilt-free binge foods. Some overweight people have a tendency to over-consume foods that are high in fat. This is mainly why they became fat in the first place. Such people are likely to consume large amounts of products that tasted like fat but did not provide its usual kilojoules. For such people, perhaps more than anyone else, we should not even consider allowing olestra into foods.

People may love guilt-free fat now, but they are unlikely to be happy if, in 20 or 30 years time, those consuming foods with fake fats turn out to have higher rates of cancer or cataracts. Such people would be justified in blaming those who allowed such products to be sold in the first place, especially when such doubts are already being publicised by concerned individuals and consumer groups.

In the United States, olestra has been approved for use in snack foods. Many dieters enjoy being able to tuck into fat-free potato crisps containing olestra, but in doing so they are ignoring warnings from groups such as the US Center for Science in the Public Interest (CSPI), a consumer health advocacy group, and others such as the American Public Health Association and the American Academy of Ophthalmology. CSPI maintains that we don't have enough evidence that olestra won't be harmful in the long term. We should surely demand of our health authorities that they give such facts more weight than the potential profits for food manufacturers who want to be able to use olestra in their products.

The National Food Authority in Australia has not yet received applications to allow olestra to be added to foods, but food manufacturers have products ready to go if they think the public will buy them. Hopefully, the Australian public will make known their feelings against such products before any are released onto the market.

## OTHER FAKE FATS

Olestra has created great interest and consternation among many nutritionists and consumer groups, but it is not the only fake fat. Others have already been approved and are widely used. Several more are in the pipeline. The older types are carbohydrate products based on starch derivatives or gums that can hold water—these types are used when some of the fat in a product is replaced by water. Others are substitutes for fat, and some newer ones are fats that have been manipulated by food technologists so that they cannot be absorbed by the body.

The food industry looks for soluble, colourless and flavourless fat substitutes carrying viscosity, coagulation, crystallisation, freezing and gelatinisation properties that are all compatible with other ingredients in the product. For example, if some of the fat is removed from a food such as margarine, it will be replaced by water, and a fat substitute will have to keep the water combined with the remaining fat so that the product retains its texture and spreadability. Some efforts at fat-reduced margarines failed because the products melted too readily and their increased water content made foods such as hot toast go soggy.

No single fat substitute works for all products. Low-fat whipped yoghurt and soft-serve ice-creams usually use a gum to hold air, rather than water, in the product. Other foods such as some types of confectionery need a poly-alcohol product that will resist the crystallisation of sugars in the product.

For many fat-reduced foods, a combination of fat substitutes is usually necessary to achieve all the characteristics desired such as creaminess, mouthfeel, processing stability, the ability to hold air and water, and bulk.

## CARBOHYDRATE-BASED FAT SUBSTITUTES

Cellulose, maltodextrins, gums, modified starches, sorbitol and other sugar alcohols, and polydextrose have all been used for some years to replace fats in some processed foods. They are useful for maintaining the structure of some products and for providing bulk, texture and mouthfeel when fat is removed.

Sugar alcohols have some sweetness as well as an ability to absorb water and act as fat substitutes in certain foods, so they are often used. They include sorbitol (additive 420), xylitol (additive 967), mannitol (additive 421), isomalt and, in some countries, maltitol and lactitol. Unlike the sugars from which they are derived, these compounds do not contribute to dental decay.

# Sorbitol

This is the oldest of the sugar alcohols, first made in 1872 from the mountain ash berry. Sorbitol also occurs naturally in cherries, plums, seaweed, apples and pears, but when it is used as a food additive for pastries, cakes and confectionery it is made in the laboratory by the hydrogenation of glucose, sucrose or starch. It contributes 16 kilojoules per gram, the same as any carbohydrate, but in the body it breaks down more slowly than sugar does. It has less than half the kilojoule level of fats. Products containing sorbitol and other sugar alcohols can cause diarrhoea if consumed in large quantities. The labels of products containing these ingredients warn that excess consumption can have a laxative effect. The high content of sorbitol in natural apple juice is a major cause of diarrhoea in young children who consume apple juice as their major liquid.

# Xylitol

This is another naturally occurring sugar alcohol that acts as a bulking agent in some fat-reduced foods. Although it can be extracted from raspberries, strawberries, some types of plums, lettuce, mushrooms, cauliflower and seaweed, xylitol is now made by hydrolysing hemicelluloses extracted from wood pulp (especially from birch trees); from the shells of almonds, coconuts or pecans; from the hulls of oats, rice or cottonseed; or from sugar cane refuse. Once hydrolysed, a sugar compound called xylose forms and this is then hydrogenated, purified and crystallised to form a white powder. Xylitol is added to foods such as ice-cream, fat-reduced chocolate and confectionery. Like sorbitol, too much can cause diarrhoea.

# Mannitol

Often used in confectionery, cake fillings and desserts, mannitol, or manna sugar as it is sometimes called, can be produced from seaweed, the wood pulp of coniferous trees, the dried exudate of the manna tree, or from various sugars. It also causes diarrhoea in large doses and makes some children nauseous. Each gram contributes about 10 kilojoules.

## Isomalt

This sugar alcohol is made from ordinary sugar, or sucrose, the glucose and fructose molecules of which are altered and joined differently, then crystallised and hydrogenated. For those interested in the chemistry, the final compound is a mixture of γ-glucopyranosyl–1 → 6-sorbitol and γ-D-glucopyranosyl–1 → 1-mannitol. It is a white, sweet-tasting crystalline powder which supposedly intensifies other flavours without having any flavour of its own. It thus acts as a substitute for sugar and fat in foods. It is used in reduced fat confectionery, drinks and ice-cream substitutes.

## Polydextrose

Formed by combining glucose, sorbitol and a small amount of citric acid, polydextrose is a carbohydrate polymer that does not taste sweet. Each gram contributes 4 kilojoules, which is one quarter the level of sugar and about one-tenth that of fats. Polydextrose is used in fat-reduced yoghurts, ice-cream and other desserts, and to replace some of the fat in fat-reduced chocolate.

One brand of polydextrose already appearing in foods is branded as Litesse™.

## Maltodextrins

These are made from various starches derived from corn, potato, rice, tapioca or a mixture of several grains, and there are dozens of different maltodextrin compounds available. In foods, they can act like a cross between sugar and starch and contribute 16 kilojoules per gram, the same level as sugars or starches. Some types can be dissolved in water and used as a fat substitute, contributing only 4 kilojoules per gram in this diluted form. Many maltodextrins are used in cakes, breads, desserts, ice-creams, fat-reduced spreads, cheese products, dips, mayonnaise, dressings and confectionery. Some types are good at binding fats, adding a creamy texture that becomes slimy if too little is used. One product derived from tapioca starch, marketed as N-Oil®, is added to some no-fat frozen desserts to replace dairy fats.

## EMULSIFIERS AND GUMS

Some or all of the fat in some foods can be replaced by emulsifiers and gums which keep water and fat evenly dispersed throughout products such as margarine, peanut butter, salad dressings and mayonnaise. They are also used to increase the quantity of air trapped in some foods such as ice-cream, or to keep products such as cakes and breads soft. Emulsifiers may be vegetable gums, compounds derived from sorbitol, or mono- and diglycerides made from vegetable oils (additives 471, 472). Lecithin (322), produced from soy beans or egg yolk, is also used as an emulsifier. Commonly used emulsifiers include polysorbates (433, 435, 436); gums derived from seaweeds such as alginic acid (400), sodium and other alginates (401–405), agar (406) and carrageenan (407); and other naturally occurring gums such as locust bean gum (408), guar gum (409), tragacanth (413), acacia (414), xanthan gum (415) and karaya gum (416).

Locust bean gum is also called carob gum or St John's bread. Chemically, it is galactomannan, and it binds water and increases the elasticity of gels made from carrageenan. It is used in processed cheese, bakery products and ice-cream.

Guar gum is also a galactomannan obtained from the seed kernel of the guar plant. It is used to thicken and stabilise foods such as sauces, ice-creams and desserts.

Tragacanth is a gum produced from a bush of the genus *Astragalus*. It swells in water to form a paste and is used as a suspending agent in no-oil salad dressings, fruit fillings and citrus beverages.

Acacia gum, or gum arabic, is exuded by wounds in the bark of *Acacia* trees. It prevents fats forming a greasy film in foods and is also used as a cloud agent in beverages.

Xanthan gum comes from the microbial fermentation of the *Xanthomonas campestris* organism. It is used in salad dressings, sauces and baked products. Karaya gum is the dried exudate from the *Sterculia urens* tree, a native of India. Because it swells in water, it is used to give body to low-fat toppings, frozen desserts and baked goods. It is also used as a denture adhesive!

## OTHER FAT SUBSTITUTES

Lita® is a new product made from protein. This time, a protein called zein, found in corn, is the raw material. Its structure resembles fat but it contributes only 6 kJ per gram, one-sixth the level of regular fats. Caprenin, another fat substitute, has some of the characteristics of chocolate but carries just 21 kJ per gram. It is made by combining glycerol with three fatty acids. Two of these are caprylic and capric acids, which have 8 and 10 carbon atoms, making them medium-chain fatty acids. The third fatty acid is behenic, a saturated fat with 22 carbon atoms made from certain varieties of rapeseed oil. Behenic acid cannot be properly absorbed by the body, so this fat substitute has a limited use.

Health authorities are having some difficulties with caprenin. Because it is made from fatty acids that occur elsewhere in nature, its manufacturers claim that it does not need special clearance as a food additive. However, caprenin's three particular fatty acids do not occur together in nature, so it may have some characteristics not yet understood.

Whenever some food additive is not absorbed, it must pass through the gastrointestinal tract. In doing so, it may either have some effect on other foods or nutrients or it may alter some types of normal, and beneficial, bacteria.

## Simplesse

A chance discovery some years ago found that fat substitutes can also be made from protein. When tiny protein particles are sheered off from whey protein (a by-product in cheese-making) during simultaneous pasteurisation and homogenisation, they form small uniform round particles. In the mouth, these tiny spherical balls formed from milk or egg protein roll around, and their mouthfeel resembles that of fat. The process is called microparticulation and the particles are so small that 50 billion could fit onto a teaspoon. Their small size gives a feeling of creaminess in the mouth. Larger particles would feel powdery or gritty. The process has been patented and a product made largely by mixing egg white and skim milk has been registered with the name

Simplesse®. It contributes only 4 kilojoules per gram, but since only small quantities are used its energy contribution is low.

Simplesse® can be used in ice-cream, and to replace the fat in sour cream, yoghurt, mayonnaise, dips and spreads; some cheese substitutes for products such as pizza have also been developed.

Some other forms of Simplesse® have been developed for bakery products, soups and products that must be heated, but the major problem for Simplesse is that it breaks down with heat so it can't be used for frying.

## DO WE NEED FAT SUBSTITUTES?

Makers of fake fats claim that their products are useful for reducing kilojoules and fat in the daily diet. Some cite the fact that saturated fats contribute to high blood cholesterol and assume that products with fat substitutes will help to lower cholesterol levels in the body. There is not proof of this.

There is no proof that fake fats help in weight reduction and there is some evidence that they do not. As these products have proliferated in countries such as the United States, the population has grown steadily fatter. The same phenomenon has occurred in Canada where almost 80 per cent of overweight women and a slightly lower percentage of overweight men use 'lite' products regularly.

Some spokespeople for the manufacturers of fake fats claim that increasing obesity is due to decreasing levels of physical activity. There is no doubt that this is correct if we look back over the last 10, 20 or 30 years. Levels of activity have not fallen, however, over the last few years since fat and sugar substitutes have been available, but the population has grown steadily fatter. There are several possible reasons for the rise in obesity: perhaps overweight people do not use fat-modified products; or perhaps using foods with fake fats induces guilt-free comfort about consuming a greater overall quantity of food. Some studies support this and show that total kilojoule intake does not decrease when people consume fat and sugar substitutes.

Foods containing fake fats are not free of kilojoules. They may have fewer kilojoules but a single-serve 50 gram pack of olestra-fried potato crisps still has 520 kilojoules, and 11 grams of olestra. The kilojoule count is less than half the level in regular crisps but is still significant, especially if you eat twice as many crisps! In such cases, there would be virtually no saving in kilojoules and a large load of olestra to pass through the intestine. If you ate other foods also containing olestra, your total daily intake could be very high.

The problem of people compensating for fake ingredients by eating larger quantities of foods is well documented in the United States. People simply eat more to make up for what they have omitted. Sugar substitutes have been well studied and there is plenty of evidence that people using them unconsciously eat more of other foods. Whether the same phenomenon occurs with fake fats is not as well documented.

While there are no proven benefits and even a small shadow of doubt hanging over some fake fats, it is difficult to justify their use. To add to their difficulties, fat substitutes cannot duplicate all the characteristics of fats. For example, a genuine ice-cream needs not only the texture and mouthfeel of cream but also its complex flavour. Even combinations of several substitutes cannot hope to match the unique richness of dairy fats. Similarly, the flavour of a good olive oil is integral to a mayonnaise or salad dressing, and no fat-free substitute can duplicate such complexity of flavour.

One of the most difficult foods for technologists to produce in fat-reduced form is cheese. It can be done to a certain extent in processed cheeses, but most true cheese lovers do not eat these products. Cheese connoisseurs doubt that anyone could ever replace the unique flavours and mouthfeel of a good cheese. They also ask why anyone would want to. We could all ask the same question.

Do we seek fat substitutes so that we can continue to stuff ourselves with vast quantities of food without getting fat? If so, they have been tried and have failed. The development of fake fats has also helped perpetuate the myth that fat is inherently bad. Some fats are. It is probably fair to say that for many adults saturated fats have little to recommend them, although they can supply a very palatable form of energy for those who *need* more kilojoules. Products such as red meat and dairy products, which are high in saturated fat, are also excellent sources of iron and calcium, nutrients that are often missing from modern diets. But all fats are not bad. Seeds, nuts, avocado, fatty fish and olive oil contain valuable and essential fats that could never be replaced with fake substitutes, and nor should they be.

Many of the foods that contain problem fats are junk foods. Replacing their fat does not give them nutritional credibility. And there is always the possibility that food additives that are totally foreign to the human gastrointestinal tract may prove to be undesirable in 20 years time. Even if the fake fats turn out to be safe, the foods containing them are still products that take the place of other more nutritious foods. If junk foods are eaten only as occasional extras, they won't cause any problems and their fats do not need to be replaced.

Other nutritious foods such as milk can easily have their fat skimmed off. Such products have been well accepted and all increases in milk sales are in this category. There is no need to manipulate these products further.

Food authorities are concerned mainly with the safety of food additives and ingredients. They do not consider such questions as whether the product is necessary, makes sense or contributes any health benefit to the nation. With olestra, many eminent scientists consider that even the safety issues are unclear. For the longest study of olestra—taking 39 weeks—the subjects were pigs.

Food technologists are trying to gain an intimate understanding of the way different fat substitutes can be combined to provide textures, mouthfeel and the processing characteristics they desire—with fewer kilojoules than fats provide. An alternative would be to abandon such pursuits and persuade people to eat the real thing, but in smaller quantities. This obviously does not suit marketing people from companies who want to produce an ever-expanding range of profitable products. It might, however, be a more justifiable use of resources.